Martial Sound

Martial Sound

Drumming Empowerment in Diasporic Chinese Kung Fu and Lion Dance

COLIN P. McGUIRE

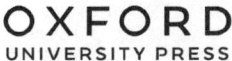

OXFORD
UNIVERSITY PRESS

OXFORD
UNIVERSITY PRESS

Oxford University Press is a department of the University of Oxford. It furthers
the University's objective of excellence in research, scholarship, and education
by publishing worldwide. Oxford is a registered trade mark of Oxford University
Press in the UK and certain other countries.

Published in the United States of America by Oxford University Press
198 Madison Avenue, New York, NY 10016, United States of America.

Library of Congress Cataloging-in-Publication Data
Names: McGuire, Colin P., author.
Title: Martial sound : drumming empowerment in diasporic Chinese kung fu and
lion dance / Colin P. McGuire.
Description: New York : Oxford University Press, 2024. |
Includes bibliographical references and index.
Identifiers: LCCN 2024034425 | ISBN 9780197775943 (paperback) |
ISBN 9780197775936 (hardback) | ISBN 9780197775950 (updf) |
ISBN 9780197775974 (other) | ISBN 9780197775967 (epub)
Subjects: LCSH: Percussion ensembles—Canada—Toronto—History and criticism. |
Military music—Canada—Toronto—History and criticism. |
Music and dance—Canada—Toronto—History. |
Music and dance—Canada—Toronto—Social aspects. |
Lion dance—Canada—Toronto—History. |
Kung fu—Canada—Toronto—History.
Classification: LCC ML3563.8.T67 M34 2024 |
DDC 791.09713/54—dc23/eng/20240806
LC record available at https://lccn.loc.gov/2024034425

DOI: 10.1093/oso/9780197775936.001.0001

Paperback printed by Marquis Book Printing, Canada
Hardback printed by Bridgeport National Bindery, Inc., United States of America

MIX
Paper | Supporting
responsible forestry
FSC
www.fsc.org   FSC® C103567

This book is dedicated to Master Paul Chan [*Chàhn Syuhyuk Sīfú*, 陳樹郁師傅] (1932–2012) and Master Jim Chan [*Chàhn Janmàhn Sīfú*, 陳振文師傅] (1929–2016), the co-founding instructors of the Hong Luck Kung Fu Club [*Hōng Lohk Móuhgún*, 康樂武舘]. Please refer to Figure 0.1 to see a photograph of them near the ends of their lives. It is my sincere hope that these pages will contribute to their goal of preserving and promoting traditional Chinese martial arts. May they rest in peace, and may their lineages endure for 10,000 years.

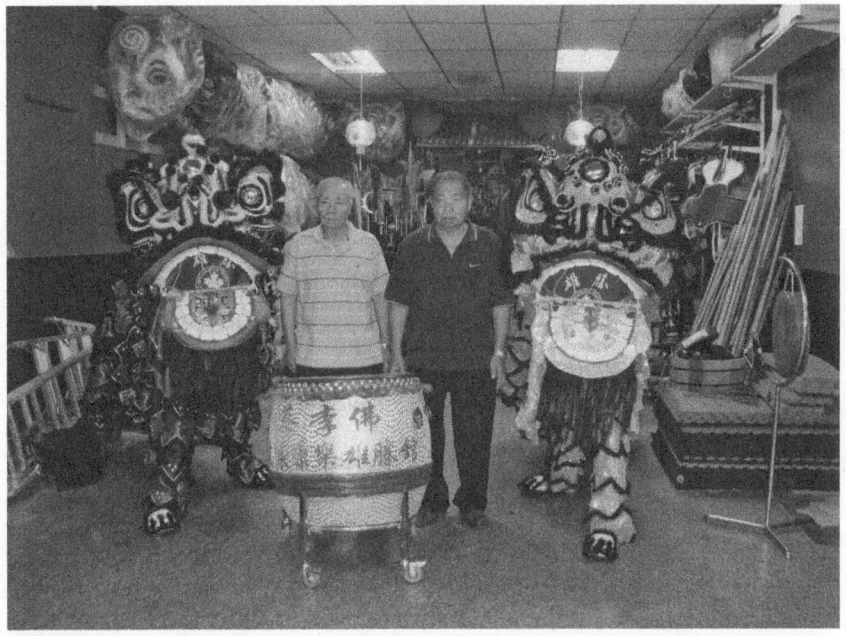

Figure 0.1 Master Jim Chan and Master Paul Chan (left and right) preparing the lion dance team for Hong Luck's fiftieth-anniversary celebrations
Credits: Colin P. McGuire

Contents

Contents

Figures

Acknowledgments

This book would not have been possible without the people who guided, supported, and encouraged me along the way. I cannot thank everyone here, but that does not mean that anyone was forgotten. Despite such excellent support, nothing is perfect; any omissions, oversights, or errors in this book are entirely my own.

When I was a PhD student at York University, my supervisor, Louise Wrazen, was always ready with thoughtful advice and constructive criticism. Her tireless efforts helped me to polish my writing, and her keen scholarship inspired me to think more clearly, carefully, and thoroughly. I also owe a debt to the other members of my dissertation committee, Mary Fogarty and Sundar Viswanathan, for their helpful comments along the way. Like every graduate student from my cohort, I am indebted to the Graduate Music Program administrator, Tere Tilban-Rios; she somehow did the work of three people and still kept her flock on track. I would also like to thank the York Centre for Asian Research for their support, with special gratitude to the ever-helpful and organized coordinator, Alicia Filipowich. After my oral defence, I received a very thorough and insightful set of edits from my external examiner, Jonathan Stock, to whom I am most grateful. As if that were not enough, he later became my mentor at University College Cork when I received a Government of Ireland Postdoctoral Fellowship to revise and augment my dissertation for this book. In the final stages before submission of the manuscript, I benefitted immensely from precise, clear, and constructive copyediting by Laura Macy.

I am very fortunate to have been supported by great people at home and in the field as well. I credit my father, Barry McGuire, for having sparked the idea to do research on music and martial arts. Thanks to my mother, Janie Campbell, for believing in me no matter what, and to Bee Sun for helping me survive learning Chinese, doing fieldwork, and writing my dissertation. My classmates, teachers, seniors, and elders at the Hong Luck Kung Fu Club accepted me into their fold and spared no effort in whipping me into shape, for which I am eternally grateful. After so many hours spent together not only training and performing, but also sharing meals and chatting, they are like another family to me. I would also like to express my appreciation for Hong Kong's Chung Chi Martial Arts Association [*Sùhnggēi Gūngfū Séh*, 崇基功夫社] and the New Asia Kung Fu Society [*Sān A Gwokseuht Wúi*, 新亞國術會]. Although I was only in Hong Kong for nine months, they packed what felt like years' worth of experience into that time. Without a Doctoral Fellowship from the Social Sciences and Humanities Research Council, I would not have been in Hong Kong in the first place. I would also like to recognize the support of the Irish Research Council in funding my postdoc, which provided the time and space to produce the manuscript for this book.

Notes on Language

I conducted fieldwork for this book in both English and Cantonese, which requires some explanation in terms of how I incorporate Chinese words into this text. Cantonese is the prestige dialect of Yue Chinese, one of the major branches of the Sinitic language family. The centre of the Yue homeland is Southern China's Guangdong Province, but it also extends into the eastern portion of the neighbouring Guangxi Zhuang Autonomous Region, northern Vietnam, and the Hong Kong and Macau Special Administrative regions. Variants of Yue predominated in North American Chinese communities from their beginnings in the mid-nineteenth century through to the twentieth; I did most of my fieldwork in just such a community. Scholars working on Chinese topics, however, have increasingly defaulted to using romanized Mandarin (a.k.a. Putonghua) in their texts because it is the national language of the People's Republic of China (PRC). Notwithstanding that the PRC promotes Mandarin as the official version of Chinese, I default to romanized Cantonese in this book to reflect the linguistic identity of my fieldwork sites in Canada and Hong Kong. My preference is for the Yale system of transliterating Cantonese in roman script, which is common among learners of Cantonese as a foreign language, despite being relatively unknown to native speakers. Both the School of Continuing Studies at the University of Toronto and the Chinese University of Hong Kong's Yale-China Chinese Language Centre used Yale romanization when I studied Cantonese with them.

Unfortunately, the situation is not as simple as picking a romanization system and sticking with it. Some naturalized Chinese words are already in good English dictionaries or are in widespread colloquial use. In such cases I will conform to what I observe to be the most common spelling— regardless of dialect or romanization system. For words that have not yet made their way into English dictionaries or common practice, but can be effectively translated, my preference is to use English translations. These will be followed by the Yale romanization and Chinese characters in brackets as necessary. In some cases, I have directly translated Chinese character-pairs and four-character phrases rather than converting them to a more elegant choice of word or expression. I have left these translations intact in the text because it marks them as being non-English through their non-idiomatic reading. It is my hope that translations will reduce the linguistic burden on readers who are unfamiliar with Chinese.

Whenever possible, I have also included Chinese characters in this book to make the text more inclusive to those who are familiar with Chinese script, but not with Cantonese or Yale romanization. Although there are significant differences in pronunciation, grammar, and vocabulary among the various Sinitic languages, they share a common character-based writing system. Written Vernacular Chinese [*Baahkwahmàhn,* 白話文] was developed in the early twentieth century based on representative contemporary literature as well as the style of Mandarin spoken in Beijing, the capital of the PRC. It gives literate Sinophones a modern, unified, text-based language—regardless of their spoken tongue. This universality is somewhat complicated by the use of two overlapping sets of ideographs: "traditional characters" [*fàahntái jih,* 繁體字] are preferred in Hong Kong, Macau, Taiwan, and the established diaspora, versus the more recently created "simplified characters" [*gáantái jih,* 簡體字] that are used in the PRC and Singapore, as well as among recent migrants from those countries. I will default to traditional characters, as preferred by my fieldwork consultants, unless otherwise specified. In the case of direct quotes from Cantonese, I will give the characters as spoken, rather than converting to Written Vernacular Chinese, and so there will be some non-standard characters. When citing sources written in simplified characters, I will leave them as written.

For Cantonese words that have no effective English translation and are not yet found in an English dictionary, I will romanize in the Yale system. These will be in italics (including diacritical tone marks), followed by Chinese characters in brackets on first occurrence. After the initial appearance of a word thus transliterated, I will use the romanized word in italics but without diacritics or characters, unless repetition would improve clarity. For the names of people, the typical order in English is given-name(s) followed by family-name, whereas in Chinese it is the reverse. In the main text, I will default to the English order if a person has a non-Chinese given-name or the Chinese order if their full name is transliterated. The Chinese ideographs for people's names (where available) will follow the Chinese order of putting the surname first, as will romanizations thereof. For place names, I will use the current officially recognized romanization.

One final consideration concerns the word *Cantonese* itself. Guangdong and its capital city Guangzhou were historically both referred to as *Canton* in English, and so the word *Cantonese* has a certain amount of ambiguity. While there are more distinct terms in Chinese, English usage typically elides the differences among several meanings. *Cantonese* can encompass the Yue language [*Yuhtyúh*, 粵語] in general, which would include various dialects. For example, Yue includes Taishanese [*Tòihsāanwá*, 台山話], a rural vernacular from Guangdong Province that once predominated in North American Chinatowns. Perhaps more often, Cantonese refers specifically to the prestige Yue dialect of Guangdong Province [*Gwóngdūngwá*, 廣東話] that originated as the vernacular in the provincial capital, Guangzhou city [*Gwóngjāuwá*, 廣 洲話]. *Cantonese* can also stand for people originating from the Greater Yue region [*Daaih Yuht yàhn*, 大粵人]. In this book, I use the word *Cantonese* specifically for the prestige dialect of Yue, not the entire language family. In a more general sense, I also use it as an ethno-linguistic moniker referring to the people and culture of the Yue language region (see Figure 0.2 for a map) and its diaspora.

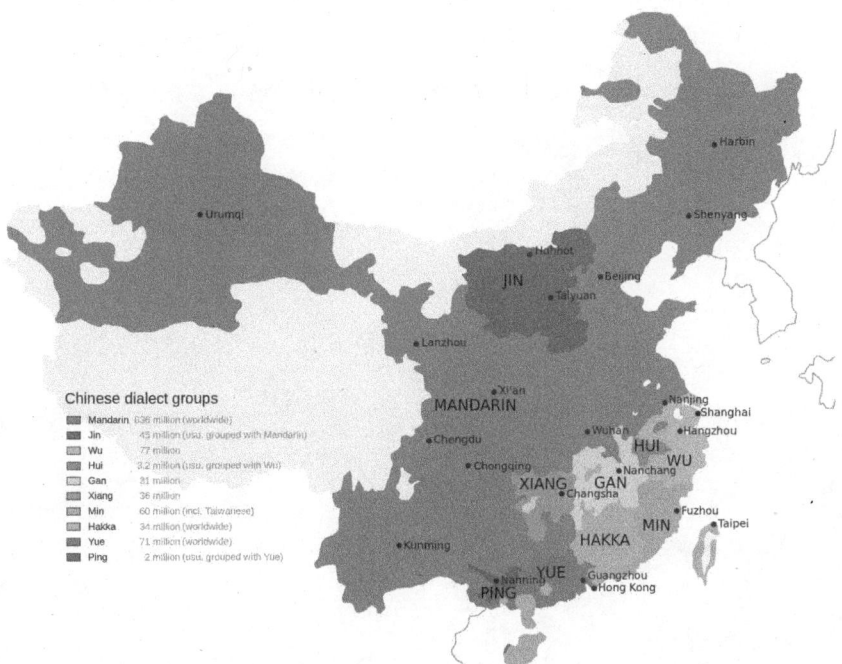

Figure 0.2 Map of Sinitic Languages, by Wyunhe, used under CC Attribution 3.0
Credits: Colin P. McGuire

Prologue

Rhythm is essential in both music and martial arts. While there are, of course, differences between the ways patterns and timing work in these two areas, there are also interesting parallels, connections, and homologies between them. Since ancient times, authors have been observing and commenting on the intersections of musical sound with fighting movements and warrior spirit. China's most famous treatise on military strategy, *The Art of War* [*Syūnjí Bīngfaat*, 孫子兵法], advised that percussion rhythms should be used to both direct and motivate armies (trans. Cleary 2003:124–127). On Chinese battlefields of yore, gongs and drums were used to signal troop movements, as well as to bolster the morale and energy of soldiers. Significantly, the Chinese character for *drum* also means "to rouse" [*gú*, 鼓]. In Plato's *The Republic*, Socrates postulated that only two types of music were fit for his ideal state (trans. Cornford 1972:85–88). One of these two encouraged bravery in times of war or danger. Socrates' ideal music deployed rhythms, words, and scales/modes thought to fuel a warrior's courage and vigour. In contemporary times, many martial arts around the world still feature musical accompaniment, including, but not limited to: Brazilian capoeira, Indonesian/Malay *pencak silat*, muay Thai, Senegalese *laamb*, Trinidadian *kalinda*, Persian *zurkhâneh*, and Sihk *gatka*. Scholars, however, have only recently begun to address the interdisciplinary field of music and martial arts, perhaps because of an underlying academic aversion to violence.

This book centres on the sound and practice of drumming, accompanied by gong and cymbal playing, in Cantonese martial arts and lion dance. Many Southern Chinese styles of "kung fu" [*gūngfū*, 功夫], as these armed and unarmed systems of hand combat are colloquially known, use a "gong and drum" [*lòhgú*, 鑼鼓] ensemble to accompany performances. Their repertoire includes rhythms for "lion dancing" [*móuhsī*, 舞獅] featuring two martial artists who animate a papier-mâché head with attached cloth body. They also have percussion repertoire for accompanying choreographed sequences of fighting movements known as "forms" [*toulouh*, 套路]. Since the end of the twentieth century, there has been an increasing amount of scholarly work on Chinese martial arts (Farrer 2011; Frank 2006; Henning 1999; Holcombe

2002; Judkins and Nielson 2015; Lorge 2012; Ma 2003; Shahar 2008; Zhou 2003). The Chinese lion dance has also received academic attention (Chan 2001; Feltham 2009; Hu 1995; Johnson 2005; Liu 2011; Slovenz 1987; Young 2006). However, until now there has been no book-length study that encompasses a balance of both kung fu and lion dancing or that integrates detailed discussion of Cantonese martial percussion in an interdisciplinary fashion.

According to my research consultants, investigating the sound, concept, and behaviour of this type of percussion separately from hand combat and lion dance would be missing the point. In fact, rather than listening to their gong and drum ensemble musically, they hear it as a type of martial art, which suggests a distinctive way of thinking about humanly organized sound. The questions of how and why they hear percussion rhythms as what I am calling *martial sound* form the refrain of this book. I undertook the primary research for this monograph during eight years of fieldwork in a Chinese Canadian kung fu club between 2008 and 2016. It is augmented by complementary research with two martial arts groups undertaken during a nine-month visit to Hong Kong in 2011/2012 and interviews conducted with female lion dancers in 2017.

Martial sound encompasses both the musical aspects of martial arts as well as ways of hearing hand combat as musicking. Distinctive combinations of timing, sound, and movement are central to the embodied being of Chinese kung fu, as well as martial arts more generally. Through considerations of embodied knowledge and heroic display, the following pages reveal martial sound's place alongside fighting skills and lion dance in Southern Chinese kung fu. Far from glorifying violence, this book engages with issues of empowerment, resistance, community, and identity in diaspora that are brought into sharp focus by a warrior ethos and are of pressing global concern in the emergent post-modern era. Despite a diverse membership and multicultural location, my consultants asserted the fundamental Chinese-ness of their practices, which leads to another research question for this book: how does the confluence of movement and sound construct a resistant identity in a diasporic community?

Prelude

The acrid smell of burning gunpowder fills the cold afternoon air as an ear-splitting cacophony of explosions echoes off the buildings lining a broad side street in Toronto's Chinatown. Loud bangs rip from a long string of firecrackers and form a ragged aural chain. But there is also the rhythmic pounding of wood beating skin, supported by pulsing crashes of metal on metal and wood on metal, which blast forth from a small-but-mighty ensemble of gong, drum, and cymbals. The unsynchronized counterpoint of explosives against percussion is exciting in its sheer sonic intensity.

Although it is the dead of winter, the Hong Luck Kung Fu Club is undeterred; Chinese Lunar New Year celebrations are getting started. The ruckus takes place in front of the club's building as its lion dance crew prepares to embark on a parade through their local Chinatown neighbourhood. A crowd of onlookers has gathered around the source of this uproar but is held at bay by a group of armed men forming a circle using staves and pole-arms to make a barrier around the performance space. Partly obscured by a cloud of smoke from the detonating firecrackers, a pair of red and black beasts are thrashing about and rending the air. Pairs of kung fu practitioners animate these Southern Chinese "lions," and their martial arts training is evident in the way they "fight" with the explosions. Their powerful stances are the base from which they launch attacks as they step, leap, crouch, and kick, all while energetically shaking the lion heads and biting at the firecrackers.

Once the pyrotechnics finish, the drummer plays a rhythmic cadence and the lion dancers respond immediately with synchronized choreography, showing both their attentiveness and their level of training. Coordinated with each other and the percussion—despite being able to see neither from beneath their costumes—the lion dancers shoot their mask-heads into the air while doing a quick cross-step before yanking the heads back down as they drop into a low squat. Having completed the opening ceremonies, the group begins its parade in earnest. Members of the kung fu club march down the sidewalk on a route that will take them around the whole neighbourhood. The percussion will stay continuous for the next four to five hours, during which time Hong Luck's lions will go door-to-door, offering short individual performances to the shops, restaurants, and associations in Chinatown.

When a multi-ethnic group performs a Cantonese custom for diverse patrons in the Chinatown of a cosmopolitan Canadian metropolis, the meanings are bound to be multiple, overlapping, and emergent. In many ways, the lion dance parade will construct Chinatown, and make a geographic place into a lived space. For some traditionally minded supporters, lion dancing at Lunar New Year is a ritual for a liminal calendrical period that will disperse negative energy and ensure their good fortune for the coming year. During the parade, Hong Luck will take extra care when lion dancing for such patrons. Increasingly, however, people see—and hear—lion dance as an entertaining spectacle that celebrates identity. Many Chinese Canadian patrons and performers will enjoy the day's lion dances as a symbol of their cultural heritage and take a more lighthearted approach to it. Non-Chinese will also be involved as a way of participating in Chinatown and supporting Hong Luck. Such participation allows a European Canadian lion dancer (like myself) or a South Asian Canadian shopkeeper to act as part of the local community. From the perspective of the kung fu club—and informed audiences—the lion dance also embodies the fighting spirit of Chinese martial arts through the vigour of movement. Fuelled by the commanding sonic presence of bellicose-sounding drumming, Hong Luck's lions will make their way through the neighbourhood, using their kung fu to create martial art that is both powerful and empowering. In fact, Chinese Canadian lion dance is all these things and more, which speaks to its enduring popularity in a land far away from where it began.

1

Entering the Field of Music and Martial Arts

Introduction

In Toronto, Canada, the Hong Luck Kung Fu Club's three-story building is a landmark in Chinatown, boasting a half-century in that neighbourhood.[1] The organization's name is emblazoned in eye-catching red-and-gold relief on the façade using both Chinese characters and English script (see Figure 1.1). After moving to Toronto in 1998, I walked past the place many times and could not help but notice the sign. On several of those occasions, I heard powerful percussion rhythms coming from inside the club. However, the large glass windows were always covered by curtains, which created a sense of mystery about the pounding beats within, as though the instruments were a secret. I knew that many Southern Chinese kung fu clubs have lion dance teams that are accompanied by an ensemble consisting of a large barrel drum complemented by a hanging gong and pairs of hand-cymbals. Nonetheless, the rhythms that I heard coming from Hong Luck seemed different: more aggressive and more powerful.

When I started a doctoral program in the fall of 2008, I had been practising the Wing Chun style of Chinese kung fu [*Wihng Chēun kyùhn*, 詠春拳] for the previous eleven years and had another fifteen years of training in a variety of other martial arts. Interested in connecting my long-time fascination with hand combat to my academic studies in ethnomusicology, I wanted to investigate the intersection of music and martial arts. I decided to explore the percussion associated with kung fu and the lion dance. It was my Wing Chun teacher, Master Henry Lo [*Lòuh Gin-hùhng Sīfú*, 盧建雄師傅], who recommended that I look to the Hong Luck Kung Fu Club as a fieldwork site,

---

[1] The Greater Toronto Area has several urban Chinatowns as well as majority Chinese ethnic suburbs. Hong Luck is located in the Spadina/Dundas neighbourhood, which is in the downtown core and is the city of Toronto's main Chinatown.

Martial Sound. Colin P. McGuire, Oxford University Press. © Oxford University Press 2024.
DOI: 10.1093/oso/9780197775936.003.0001

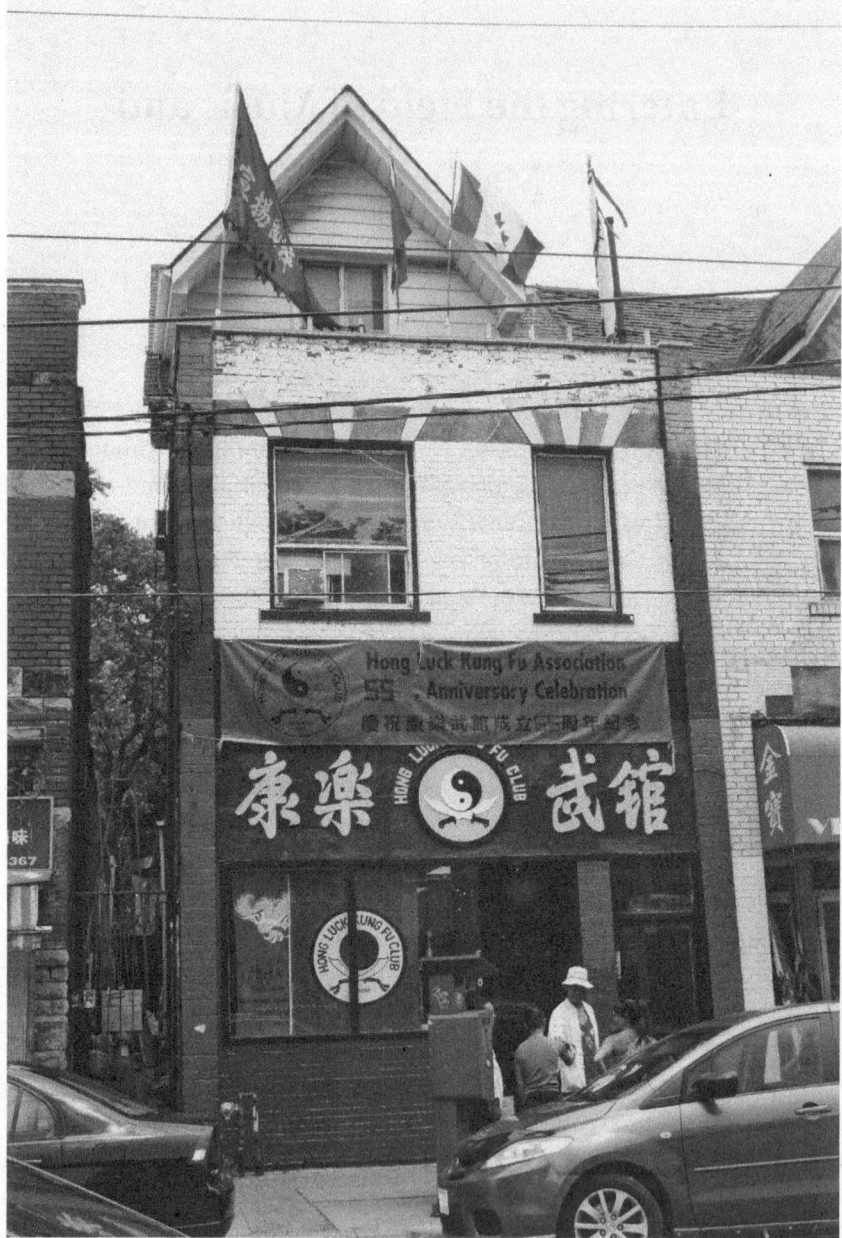

Figure 1.1 Hong Luck's building at 548 Dundas St. West
Credits: Colin P. McGuire

saying they were not only the most "traditional," but had the best drummers in the Greater Toronto Area (GTA). The group also had a well-established reputation in the local martial arts scene, and so I decided to explore the possibility of doing fieldwork there.

I walked into Hong Luck for the first time on a Tuesday night in early September 2008. It was shortly before the start of a beginner class, and several students were already on the floor stretching, shadowboxing, or chatting. I was pleased to note that the back of the training hall was lined with the big masks used for lion dancing, and I could see several drums sitting among the racks of weapons and miscellaneous pieces of training equipment. The gritty atmosphere was impressive; everything in the place looked well worn, as though from hard use. A teacher greeted me when I came in and casually fielded my questions. He barely raised an eyebrow when I told him that I was looking to do research at Hong Luck, which surprised me. I later learned that the club's street-level location attracts a lot of attention from passers-by, but few people who show interest actually join up—even fewer persevere longer than a month or two. The teacher answered my initial queries about drumming, telling me that the best way to understand it would be by learning to do it myself. He also informed me that—just like everybody else—I would have to start with basic training in Hong Luck's martial arts. The privilege of learning anything else is based on students' effort in, dedication to, and progress with kung fu. The teacher invited me to watch the class that night, and then I filled out some forms, bought a uniform (logo tee-shirt and black cotton waist sash), paid a registration fee, and became a de jure member of the club.

As I discovered upon my initial inquiry, Hong Luck's drummers understand their beats through drumming. While that may sound like a circular explanation, a deeper examination reveals the embodied knowledge that becomes audile in practice. I soon discovered that Hong Luck's drumming is, to borrow a phrase from Timothy Rice (2003), *learned but not taught*; there is no formal curriculum for the percussion. Instead, the pedagogical environment bears similarities to what Jonathan Stock has observed about Shanghainese opera apprenticeship in the early twentieth century, where singing "was not so much taught to new apprentices as learned by them" through immersion and observation (Stock 2002: 22). At Hong Luck, prospective drummers first become familiar with the rhythms through lion dancing, which is accompanied by the percussion in both training and performance. Similarly, learners start experiencing the percussion patterns for accompanying choreographed martial arts demonstrations through performing such kung fu demos themselves. It is up to would-be drummers, however, to translate their embodied knowledge onto the drum. Similarly, students learn lion dance through martial arts. The lion dance relies on the footwork of Hong Luck's hand combat system, and even the ability of the percussionists and lion dancers to synchronize with each other is thought to be acquired through drilling fighting techniques. Hong Luck builds drumming on a foundation of lion dance, and lion dance is undergirded by martial arts. All the full-fledged drummers I spoke with at Hong Luck confirmed this semi-autodidactic transmission process; they surely received comments and criticism from members of their community of practice but essentially had to teach themselves to drum based on their embodied experience with the rhythms.

The brief interaction that first night not only initiated my fieldwork researching the connections between music and martial arts, but also helped to establish an epistemology and methodology. My path to becoming a drummer and understanding the drum rhythms was laid out for me by the transmission process. I would need to become proficient in an unfamiliar style of kung fu as well as learn to lion dance. Only then could my own body become a fieldwork site for the embodied knowledge that undergirds this drumming, but is only incompletely verbalized by practitioners. During eight years of study, training, performing, and eventually teaching at Hong Luck (2008–2016), I was the only person who went all the way through from neophyte to regular drum performer. Nonetheless, there were established and prospective drummers around who provided the essential sociocultural context, and intersubjectively anchored the transmission process. I was fortunate to have had two main lion dance teachers and to have become a disciple of one of the club's two founding masters, but even non-drumming members contributed to my development. More often than not, they showed me what was important rather than told me. Given the relatively limited verbal discourse about music at Hong Luck, the effort to externalize my own embodied experience of drumming is a key aspect of this book, thus making the research a form of performance ethnography. At the same time, I also provide thick description of teaching, learning, and performing martial arts, lion dancing, and percussion that is based on participant observation and ongoing discussions with Hong Luck members. I will return to the issues raised by these methods shortly, but first I shall introduce my findings.

Studying martial arts to learn percussion in the context of a Chinese Canadian kung fu club gradually brought three key themes into focus: empowerment, community, and identity. These themes are important components in the ways that drumming intersects meaningfully with martial arts in the life-worlds of Hong Luck members and their patrons. A bit of history will help illustrate this point. Despite having established communities early in Canada's history (1858), migrants from China and their descendants have remained a minority.[2] They have historically struggled for acceptance from European Canadians, who have been both more numerous and politically dominant. Put plainly, Chinese Canadians have long suffered racial discrimination as a result of white supremacy (Gillborn 2006). Their tribulations have had a lasting effect on Chinatown communities, particularly in the form of mutual-aid associations as central social institutions. Hong Luck was founded in 1961 as just such an association, which was during an era when ethnically motivated violence was still all too common. On the one hand, the founding masters taught self-defence skills to their local Chinese Canadian community, so that people could resist physical racism. On the other, Hong Luck has been open to non-Chinese Canadians since its early days, thus using kung fu strategically to build bridges between Chinatown and other communities. The club has also explicitly sought to preserve and promote Chinese culture in Canada through martial arts, lion dance, and percussion, which extends the idea of self-defence to protecting values, meanings, and beliefs. Combining defence of self and culture with community building is crucial to the way that Hong Luck has contributed to the ongoing (re)construction of Chinese identity in diaspora.

This book presents an ethnography of Hong Luck's martial drumming and argues that these sounds auralize an empowered community identity. The realities of lived experience in a multicultural and multigenerational context, however, are not as neat and tidy as my thesis might suggest. Hong Luck contains, connects, and borders on a variety of communities. The identities of Hong Luck members and patrons are neither singular nor fixed, but rather they are multiple, intersecting, dynamic, emergent, negotiated, and contested. Despite these noisy communities and boisterous identities, the club also fosters a remarkably inclusive solidarity. What I am pursuing here is not a minutely qualified set of sub-identities as points of stabilization; I seek an understanding of the processes and relationships that are at

---

[2] The first Chinese people in Canada arrived on the West Coast in 1788. They were brought over by Captain John Meares to work as shipbuilders, but did not establish a permanent settlement. Chinese migration to Canada began in earnest with the gold rush of the 1850s.

work. I contend that Hong Luck inculcates discourses of Chinese-ness and resistance to oppression through their transmission process. In performance, the percussion rhythms that accompany kung fu demonstrations and lion dancing act as a catalyst for manifesting this embodied knowledge to audiences. Given that practitioners stress the Chinese-ness of their arts, the diverse membership and multicultural context point towards a flexible ontology of what it means to be Chinese in diaspora. Hong Luck is a producer of sonic and bodily culture for overseas Chinese, Canadian-born Chinese, and non-Chinese Canadians alike, while also negotiating the variety of subject positions, stances, and identities the practitioners carry with them before, during, and after training. As the club navigates its sixth decade, it is also a product of the processes that have been transmitting a specifically Cantonese, martial way of being-in-the-world within the pressure cooker of a cosmopolitan metropolis. The rest of this chapter will provide an overview description of Hong Luck's practices, establish a framework for thinking about martial sound, and engage with issues of research methodology.

Practices of the Hong Luck Kung Fu Club

The combination of fighting skills, lion dancing, and percussion rhythms at my primary fieldwork site draws together several of the major styles of Southern Chinese martial arts. As a result, I consider Hong Luck to be a school of kung fu not only in the sense of a teaching institution, but also as a distinct lineage. Over the course of the forty-seven years before I started training there in 2008, successive generations of students learned a group of related but distinct types of Southern Chinese martial arts. Different styles had priority at different points in the club's history according to the evolving practice of head and assistant instructors, as well as visiting masters. Several senior Hong Luck members have remarked to me that they feel their lineage is more than the sum of its parts; it is a style unto itself. While practitioners still differentiated between the stylistic origins of choreographed sets or characteristic techniques from the constituent hand-combat systems, my consultants also reflected on the considerable cross-influence between the individual styles. Hong Luck's syncretism is most evident in three areas: combat, lion dance, and percussion. Practitioners rarely differentiated between the stylistic origins of their fighting, dancing, or musicking, but rather experienced and applied them as integrated within the school's lineage. I will now provide a brief introduction to the club and its main styles, although I reserve more detailed information for Chapter 2.

Master Paul Chan and Master Jim Chan co-founded the Hong Luck Kung Fu Club in 1961 as a martial arts association. Despite sharing a surname and both hailing from Taishan county in Guangdong Province, China, the founders met for the first time in Toronto. They originally began training with a group of eleven associates in improvised locations, such as the basements and backrooms of the Chinese restaurants where the two co-founders worked. The club eventually purchased a building located at 548 Dundas Street West, where it has remained since 1968. While the Hung Gar style of kung fu [*Hùhng Gā kyùhn*, 洪家拳] played a more important role in the early days, the two main systems practised at Hong Luck during my fieldwork were Choi Lee Fut [*Choi Léih Faht kyùhn*, 蔡李佛拳] and Do Pi [*Douh paai*, 道派], both of which are hybrid styles synthesized in the nineteenth and early twentieth centuries from older types of Southern Chinese martial arts. In general, all these kung fu systems can be described as "long-bridge wide-horse" [*chèuhng kìuh daaih máah*, 長橋大馬] types of "Southern boxing" [*nàahm kyùhn*, 南拳]. These two idiomatic expressions are shorthand ways of referring to dichotomies in Chinese martial arts between strategic preferences for long-range versus short-range combat, as well as the wide stable stances favoured in the South versus the more acrobatic footwork of the North. In Chapter 2, I will address the individual histories of Choi Lee Fut and Do Pi, as well as that of Hong Luck, but throughout the rest of the book I will only differentiate these constituent kung fu styles if there is something that requires highlighting.

The club's basic hand-combat curriculum consists of stances, stepping, punches, kicks, and blocks, as well as several choreographed sets (a.k.a. forms) that combine discrete techniques and movements into sequences. This training program does not constitute a rigid syllabus, so it has varied over time and still depends on who is teaching any given class. During my fieldwork, the head instructor only taught one class per week to a group of advanced students, while the other six weekly classes where each led by a different assistant instructor. In the thrice-weekly beginner classes, between five and fifteen students would stand in rows and drill their techniques in time with their teacher's counting, but they did so as a form of shadowboxing (i.e., without contacting anyone or anything). Less frequently, there was light-contact partner training and full-power striking of focus pads or hanging sand bags. Occasionally, beginner students learned brief breathing meditations, did general fitness exercises like jogging and stretching, or got to try out simple joint locks on each other. Learners could only join intermediate and advanced classes upon the invitation or nomination of an instructor. Beginners had to demonstrate an adequate grasp of the fundamentals, a command of the basic choreographed forms, and sufficient physical conditioning before they got to learn weapons forms, more sophisticated empty-hand forms, lion dance, percussion, or sparring applications. The multiple purposes that Hong Luck ascribes to martial arts include self-defence, competition, performance, fitness, health, spirituality, and wellness, as well as preserving and promoting Chinese culture.

Lion dance is an intermediate class and the only session that regularly includes percussion; it is where people learn to play the instruments. The costume consists of a puppet-like mask with attached cloth cape, which a pair of performers animate in the roles of head and tail, respectively. The head is large enough to cover the front performer's whole upper torso, and it has moveable mouth, eyes, and ears. The cape forms the body as it drapes over the bent back of the performer in the rear. At Hong Luck, my teachers taught in English and called the instruments by their English names, although I will include the Chinese words used by the Cantonese-speaking elders for reference. The standard lion dance percussion ensemble consists of a membranophone, a metallophone, and a pair or more of metal idiophones: a large, single-headed, barrel "drum" [*gú*, 鼓] beaten with two short, stubby, wooden sticks; a smallish, flat-faced, hanging "gong" [*lòh*, 鑼] that is struck with a short, knobbed, wooden stick; and one or more pairs of small to medium "cymbals" (spoken onomatopoeically as *chā* [鑔] but rendered in formal speech and writing as *baht* [鈸]) that are played by holding a central knob and striking them together concussively (see Figure 1.2). Lion dance functions like kung fu in terms of being a combination of martial, performative, physical, and cultural elements, but it also includes a higher degree of ritual symbolism. Traditionally, a lion's fearsome appearance and the forceful percussion are believed to exorcise bad energy. At the same time, lions are lucky, because when they "eat" the food provided by patrons, they spit it back out to symbolically spread good fortune, which I will explain more fully in Chapter 2.

The ideal Hong Luck practitioner would be able to perform choreographed forms, fight, lion dance, play the instruments, and teach. In practice, however, individual people have their own interests and talents, so it is common for members to focus on only one or two areas. As compared to the ranking

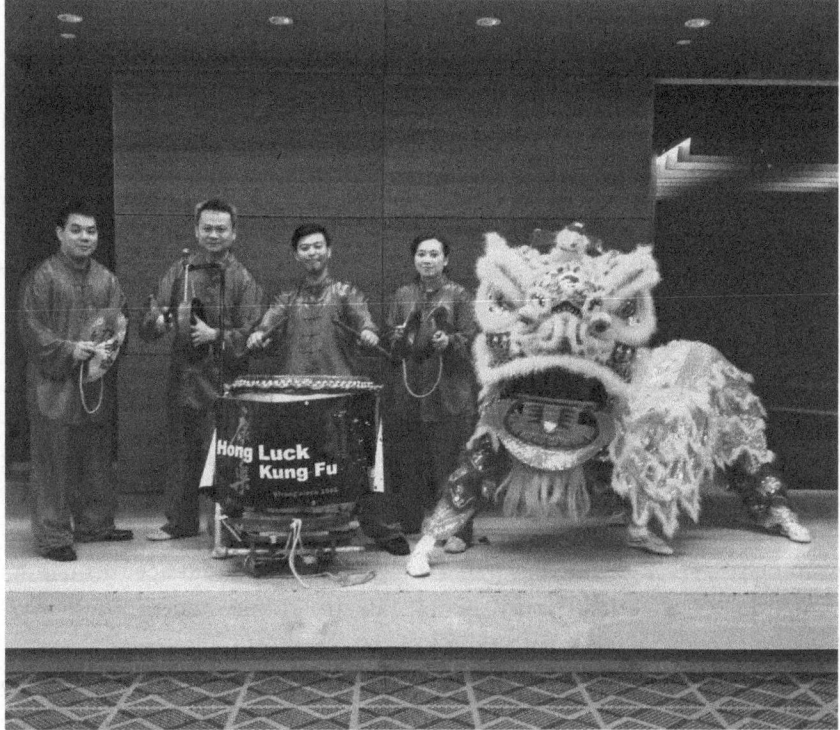

Figure 1.2 Hong Luck lion dance team with instruments
Credits: Colin P. McGuire

systems that grew out of modernization efforts in Japanese martial arts like judo and karate, there have traditionally been no black belts in Chinese martial arts. Instead, kung fu is more like a path where progress is measured in hours of hard work and years of seniority leading towards the ever-elusive goal of mastery; the journey is more important than the goal because, somewhat paradoxically, the goal is unattainable. Or as Master Jim once told me with a twinkle in his eye during an impromptu evaluation, "your kung fu eighty, maybe ninety percent. Hundred percent impossible, but keep practise anyway!"[3]

---

[3] Most of my conversations with Master Jim were in Cantonese, but he sometimes switched to broken English for emphasis or so that other students who did not speak Chinese could overhear and understand.

Kung Fu and Martial Sound

Now, I need to clear up two possible misconceptions. Firstly, the literal meaning of the term *kung fu* in Modern Standard Chinese is "skill achieved through time and effort," not martial arts. Or as, several martial arts masters have explained to me, one needs to be willing to suffer to achieve skill. The English usage of *kung fu* to refer to Chinese hand-combat systems most likely stems from the way Cantonese speakers colloquially prefer *gūng fū* [功夫] over the more formal and literal term for "martial arts" [*móuhseuht*, 武術] (Judkins 2014). In contrast, my Mandarin teachers at York University taught me to privilege the "proper" version in both speech and writing. The linguistic borrowing of kung fu to mean Chinese martial arts in English is not surprising given that Cantonese-speaking Hong Kong was under British rule from the mid-nineteenth century until 1997 (apart from Japanese occupation during WWII). While small in geographic size, Hong Kong has had a huge worldwide influence through its film industry, affecting the way people talk and think about Chinese martial arts.

The idea of kung fu as proficiency refined by practice is as applicable to cooking or painting as it is to hand combat. The hallmarks of kung fu are literally persistence, discipline, and determination; these qualities are pertinent to many forms of skilled practice. For example, when I visited Shanghai for a conference in 2013, I passed by a tea shop that was slightly off the beaten path for tourists. After looking around, I asked the proprietor in my halting Mandarin if I could sample his wares before buying. He grabbed some of the oolong tea that I pointed at, threw the leaves into a glass, poured water on it from a thermos, and handed it to me. He appeared amused as I awkwardly attempted to sniff and taste the scalding hot liquid that was becoming bitter as it cooled. I then asked him what his favourite was, and he replied kung fu tea, which is a process and not a varietal. The shopkeeper seated me at a rickety table in the back of his shop and proceeded with a more elaborate preparation involving a careful measure of tea leaves in a small earthenware teapot and two separate rounds of hot water, the first of which he quickly discarded. The resulting infusion that he poured into a cup for me was ready to drink as well as both aromatic and sweet. Evidently, skill in preparation was as important as the quality of the ingredients—if not more so. I purchased some of the tea that I sampled, and, after returning to Canada, I tried many times to copy his method. Although my results improved with practice, I was never able to achieve as fine a brew as the shopkeeper. Apparently, my tea kung fu still needs work.

The second possible misconception is that the percussion rhythms of Cantonese martial arts and lion dance are "music." As it turns out, practitioners do not think of them that way. For example, my aforementioned Wing Chun teacher, Master Henry Lo, seemed genuinely confused when I embarked on my doctoral studies and told him that I was planning on researching Chinese gong and drum music. He told me it was "just" drumming and not really music at all, to which he added that it was missing melody. In Hong Kong, the members of the New Asia Kung Fu Society told me that doing "ethnomusicology" [màhnjuhk yāmngohk hohk, 民族音樂學] on this percussion did not make sense as it was simply "drum beats" [gú dím, 鼓點], not "music" [yāmngohk, 音樂], per se. At Hong Luck, a senior drummer told me that he does not consider himself a musician or capable of playing music because he "only" knows how to drum. Drumming may not be music, but it is considered one of the most advanced skills in kung fu, because hand combat and lion dance training are both prerequisites for it. In fact, practitioners do not separate these areas, but rather they take them all as coextensive aspects of the martial arts—broadly considered. Drummers hone their craft as drum kung fu in both the literal sense of skill achieved through hard work over time and the colloquial meaning of martial arts.

The comments made by my interlocutors claiming their percussion tradition is not actually music deserve an explanation in terms of why an ethnomusicologist like myself might be studying it. Fellow ethnomusicologists may find some of this explanation and literature survey redundant, and I invite them to gloss over it, but this book is directed at an interdisciplinary audience who would benefit from such positioning. On a basic level, gong and drum beats have musical qualities such as rhythm patterns and regular tempos. They are also played on percussion instruments that could be considered musical instruments in other contexts. Notwithstanding that the word *ethnomusicology* breaks down to culture-music-study, John Blacking inclusively defined its purview as humanly organized sound (1973). In writing about the concept of music, Bruno Nettl suggested that ethnomusicologists may be a bit gluttonous because they "as a group take a broad view, accepting everything conceivable into their scope of study" (2005: 25). He went on to write that this inclusivity seeks to avoid ethnocentrism but is only partially successful. The Western origin of ethnomusicology means that disciplinary terminology will not always line up with definitions in other languages and cultures. For example, the difficult position of musical activity in Islam leads to Koranic cantillation not being considered music, which shelters it from being forbidden under some interpretations of Islamic law (al Faruqi 1985). Nonetheless, this type of religious singing can be described musically (al Faruqi 1978). Similarly, the Inuit throat-game *katajjaq* is played as a vocal competition, but scholars have transcribed it in music notation to compare it to other circumpolar practices like shamanic songs in Siberia (Nattiez 1999). Ethnomusicology has specialized tools for the description and analysis of humanly organized sound; these tools can be applied to a variety of phenomena regardless of culturally constructed notions surrounding what music is or is not.

The non-music concept of drumming held by my research consultants has important interpretive possibilities. To align my discourse with these opportunities, I will take up three strategies. First, I will avoid labelling kung fu and lion dance percussion beats as music. This move is not merely semantic, but rather mitigates a form of symbolic violence via the imposition of a hegemonic category. Second, I will bracket any questions about the ontology of music that this discussion may raise, and defer to Christopher Small's (1998) well-known concept of *musicking*. Gong and drum beats may not be music (whatever that is), but to paraphrase Small, the act of taking part, in any capacity, in a performance of humanly organized sound is *to music*. This move creates space for ethnomusicological investigations of gong and drum performances, whether or not they are music. It also opens the possibility of discussing martial arts movements as musicking, which will help me to analyze the rhythm of combat that is manifested in patterns of attack and defence. Fortunately, none of my consultants insisted on a non-musical ontology of gong and drum rhythms, nor were they offended by referring to their percussion rhythms as music. My main drumming mentor agreed with my assertion that the beats are musical, even if they are not "really" music, so talking about musicking is an apt theoretical move.

As a third strategy for dealing with non-music musicking, I am introducing a new way of thinking about the sonic aspects of martial arts. I propose the term *martial sound* to refer to the percussion rhythms of kung fu and lion dance. More broadly, martial sound is any sonic material that is humanly organized in time, and whose presence is a component of training, competition, combat, ritual, and/or performance in any type of martial art whatsoever. I am purposefully casting a wide net with this term to encompass not only instruments like the gong and drum of kung fu, but also the rhythm of combat. In martial arts, combative rhythms are manifested, inter alia, in the thud of strikes landing or being defended, the whizz of armed or unarmed attacks cutting through the air, the clash of weapons against each other, the patter of footwork, and the snap of clothing from vigorous martial motion. I further include self-accompanying noises like vocalizations, breathing, slaps, claps, and stomps that martial artists manifest in practising, performing, and fighting, as well as the rhythms beat out by them on training equipment like punching bags, focus pads, and wooden dummies. Music that is actually thought of as music could also be martial sound when it is coextensive with martial arts, as with the musical bow-driven singing of Brazilian capoeira. The interface of sonic and kinetic is central to my concept of martial sound, but it need not be physical. Music in martial arts films becomes martial sound through co-presence on screen. The intertextual association between sound and hand combat can become so engrained through repeated co-presentation that a piece of music can retain its martial arts associations off-screen. For example, the theme song of a Southern Chinese martial arts master named Wong Fei-hung has been used in over one hundred Hong Kong films and TV shows. Its kung fu associations with righteous valor have empowered its use as martial sound in various political protests (McGuire 2018). Another extension of the idea is found in imagined acoustic textures written into the action of nineteenth-century Chinese martial arts novels through onomatopoeic, environmental, and dialect-based "sounds rising from the paper," as documented by literature scholar Paize Keulemans (2014). At the limit, one might even apply the concept to situations where there is no prima facie connection between music and martial art, as with pop tunes blasting in a kickboxing gym. Put another way, martial sound is the soundscape of human combative being-in-the-world (cf. Schafer 1993).

Thinking of kung fu percussion in terms of martial sound, rather than as music, draws on what sound-studies scholar Jonathan Sterne calls *sonic imaginations* (2012). This approach seeks to maintain a position that is both inside a sound culture and simultaneously outside of it. Sterne suggests that sonic imaginations facilitate work that represents sound while recognizing that any re-presentation is an opportunity for reflexive reconfiguration that can reveal previously unexamined qualities, functions, and meanings. Martial sound is also related to other works in sound studies on combat, while remaining distinct from them. In his book investigating the total sonic experience of wartime Iraq, Martin Daughtry proposes the term *belliphonic* to encompass everything from explosives, gunfire, fighter jets, armoured vehicles, and power generators to propaganda blasting out of loudspeakers and music in soldiers' headphones (2015: 3–4). In a similar vein, Steve Goodman (2010) has written about sonic warfare as the physicality of sound waves deployed through immersive environments to produce what he calls an *affective tonality* of fear and dread. His discussion focuses on the politics of frequency, but encompasses a "battlefield" that includes not only military and commercial applications, but also musical and artistic ones. Martial sound inhabits a similar audio-conceptual space as belliphonic and sonic warfare, but is more anachronistic in its connection to hand combat. While modern technology is central to both Daughtry and Goodman's discussions, it is peripheral to my conception of martial sound.

A goal of coining the term *martial sound* is to engage in theoretical conversations both within and beyond my home discipline of music. Ethnomusicology has absorbed theory from other areas of the social sciences and humanities, but ethnomusicological theory has tended to have less impact outside its home discipline (Rice 2010). For example, the influential idea that culture can be "read" as "text" (Geertz 1973) borrows from literary criticism and phenomenology to inform interpretive ethnography. Briefly, philosopher Paul Ricoeur (1984) explains how meaningful action can be analyzed through a hermeneutic arc whereby textual structure reveals a world that one can appropriate through interpretive understanding. The other direction of Ricoeur's hermeneutic arc is also significant, where meaningful action is pre-understood without the need for structural analysis or interpretation (Rice 1994). In this case, text in the form of embodied meaning is already understood through practice, but analysis and interpretation lead to an enriched understanding. As useful as the idea of cultural textuality may be, Jeff Titon has proposed "that we stand Ricoeur on his head, that meaningful actions be experienced as music, not read as text" (2008 [1997]: 28–29). In the case of martial arts, hearing hand combat as musicking allows the interpretation of choreomusical relationships between sound and movement that are recalcitrant to linguistic models of text. As I will explain later in the book, the rhythm of combat has occasionally been addressed by practitioners (Lee 1975; Miyamoto 1982 [1645]), but not with the broadness of martial sound. An ethnomusicological approach to hearing combative behaviour not only clarifies its musical qualities, but also opens unexplored meanings to analysis. In the next section, I expand on my way of thinking about percussion in and as martial arts.

Martial Arts as Blurred Genres

Consistent with other scholarly interest in martial arts that involve musicking, I draw on Clifford Geertz's (1980) work as a helpful way of theorizing complex combinations of fighting skills, martial sound, and dance. Geertz originally used the term *blurred genre* in regard to the social sciences and humanities, where contemporary writing often elides differences between formerly separate academic disciplines. His idea was picked up by anthropologists studying the Brazilian dance-fight-game capoeira because of the way music and movement are interwoven through the variable dynamics of playing, competing, fighting, dancing, and performing (Lewis 1992; Downey 2002, 2005). Similarly, the editors of *The Fighting Art of Pencak Silat and Its Music: From Southeast Asian Village to Global Movement* also invoke the idea of blurred genre in the book's introduction (Paetzold and Mason 2016). Their volume includes not only music and martial arts in Southeast Asia, but also theatre and dance forms that incorporate techniques, postures, and gestures from local hand-combat styles, which shows how an integrated approach can reveal layers of martial meaning and symbolism that might otherwise be missed in ethnomusicology and/or ethnochoreology. A non-martial example of the blurred genre phenomenon would be the imbrication of sound and movement in West African polyrhythms, where dancing completes drum patterns; addressing only the so-called music itself would make little sense (Chernoff 1979).

I am advocating for a theory of martial arts as a blurred genre that includes all the coextensive physical, social, and cultural ways that people emulate, practise, represent, perform, strategize, prepare for, compete in, and face violence, whether it be through hand combat or through sound and movement. More briefly, I consider martial arts to be ways of addressing violence, which may or may not involve engaging in physical combat. In a way, this proposition moves in the direction of an older Chinese term for "martial arts" [*móuhngaih*, 武藝] that "emphasizes the broader humanistic aspects of these arts" (Henning 2006: 12), rather than the circumscribed techniques of fighting. However, as soon as one moves to define boundaries—even blurry ones—exceptions arise. For example, modern warfare is primarily the purview of large-scale, professional, armed forces who focus on the use of advanced weaponry. The technology-based methods and strategies of contemporary militaries are therefore outside the physio-socio-cultural purview of the martial arts that I am proposing. Nonetheless, soldiers may still train in martial arts, such as the United States Marine Corps Martial Arts Program (MCMAP). Moreover, armies continue to employ martial sound, such as the bagpipe bands found in many Highland regiments. The idea of martial arts as blurred genre gets at how they are constituted along a wide continuum of efficacy and entertainment (Farrer 2015, further to Schechner 1974). Drawing hard genre boundaries between "real" martial arts versus combat-dance, stage fighting, and/or martial sound runs the risk of turning a fertile continuum into a limiting opposition.

Few people would likely question whether an East Asian style of hand combat like Chinese kung fu is a martial art, but grouping percussion beats and lion dance under that designation may be slightly more contentious. In the recently established inter-discipline of martial arts studies (and its prototypes), scholars have strived to define their object of research in a way that can encompass a diverse range of practices as well as allow an equally diverse set of methods (for early examples, see: Bolelli 2003; Green 2001; Jones 2002b). The focus of scholarly attention has largely been on *martial* technique as the central characteristic, with the *art* component being more about skill than aesthetics. A working consensus takes the term *martial arts* as the overarching category for all manner of skilled human combative behaviour, whether the actual practice centres on combat, competition, sport, self-defence, performance, education, fitness, self-cultivation, meditation, ritual, imagination, or some combination thereof. Such a definition works towards dismantling a lingering Orientalism that limits martial arts to being "traditional" East Asian forms of self-defence, such as: judo, karate, kung fu, and taekwondo. Combat sports like Greco-Roman wrestling, self-defence systems like Israeli *krav maga*, fight-dances like *pencak silat seni* from West Java, and moving meditations like the simplified Beijing twenty-four-posture tai chi form would thus all fall under the martial arts designation—broadly considered.

Debates about defining martial arts have become more nuanced since the launch in 2015 of an open-access peer-reviewed journal called *Martial Arts Studies*. Sixt Wetzler (2015), a curator at the German Blade Museum, has made a convincing argument for defining martial arts not by what they are, but rather through a poly-systems approach to the recurrent dimensions of meaning that they participate in, the phenomena that actualize those meanings, and the historicity of the phenomena.[4] He adds a helpful caveat

---

[4] Wetzler's five initial dimensions of meaning include, but are not limited to: preparation for violent conflict, play and competitive sports, performance, transcendent goals, and health care

on the difficulty of determining the historical origins of many types of combative movement—whether they arose in combat, dance, drama, ritual,
performance, or imagination—hence preventing a dogma of "realism"
from ossifying the discussion. Wetzler's descriptive approach was meant to
foster open-mindedness about martial arts studies, which helped Benjamin
Judkins (2016) to analyze the recently invented practice of lightsaber
combat (à la *Star Wars* films) as a martial art. While Wetzler's approach is
inclusive, it is still predicated on a minimal definition of martial arts that is
based on "methods for the wide continuum of physical struggle" (Wetzler
2015: 24, further to Lorge 2012). I am intervening in the debate to desta-
bilize the "physical struggle" paradigm before the identity of martial arts
becomes too circumscribed to reach its potential as a truly interdisciplinary
field of study.

Regarding definitions, cultural-studies scholar Paul Bowman (2016) has
cautioned against the spectre of naïve scientism that lurks in the effort to
concretely demarcate entities that are always-already emergent, manifold,
and constructed, arguing instead that scholars need to put theory first. In a
poststructuralist mode, Bowman proposes that it is more productive to focus
on theorizing "how discourses and identities are constituted, and the logics
of their processes of establishment, stabilization, interaction, transformation, and dissolution" (2016: 18). I suggest that an excessive focus on physical
combat could prematurely discount some practices from consideration as
martial arts. Viewed from my perspective in writing this book, martial sound
is as much a part of some types of kung fu as fighting skills are. Following
Bowman, what is needed is a theory of how hand combat relates to practices
like music, dance, or theatre, as well as how such artistic practices can be
constituted as martial arts when they are not conventionally considered to
be combative.

I propose that thinking of martial arts in terms of performance both
facilitates the investigation of their non-combative aspects and underscores
how the training of fighting skills is performative. Some conceptions of the
martial arts are victim to a conceit that privileges physical struggle over all
other forms of martial behaviour, as though the only way to deal with violence was through actual hand combat. As an antidote to such narrow

(2015: 26). His classes of phenomena are: the body, movement/technique, tactics/concepts,
weapons/materiality, media representation, teaching methodology/learning process, myths/philos-
ophy, social structures, and wider cultural context (2015: 26–28).

conceptualizations, I point to the work of ethnographer and actor-trainer Phillip Zarrilli, who coined the term *heroic display ethos*: "that collective set of behaviors, expected actions, and principles or codes of conduct that ideally guide and are displayed by a hero, and are the subject of many traditional ballads or epics where seemingly superhuman heroes display bravery, courage, and valor in the face of death" (2010: 606; see also Klens-Bigman 2002, 2007). Of course, culturally constructed ways of martial being-in-the-world also allow for anti-heroes, like the roguish ideal embodied in capoeira's quality of *malícia* or cunning trickery (Diaz 2017). The heroic-display ethos gets at the ways that martial arts in the modern world are always-already institutional, constructed, and mediatized so that representation—and performance—are as important as application (Bowman 2015). The work of Griffith Rollefson (2017) provides a further example of the possibilities that arise from thinking about martial arts as more than just hand combat. He has written about rap music as a metaphysical (not metaphorical) martial art, noting how deep-rooted imagery within the genre weaponizes lyrics for self-defence. Hip-hop music can thus be heard as applying martial sound through what Rollefson calls *s/wordplay* (conflating swordplay with wordplay), where lyrical flows launch attacks against both literal and symbolic violence.

In sum, the real question is not "what are martial arts?" but rather, "what can we productively study as martial arts?" The claims of my research consultants inspire my argument. They maintained that their lion dancing and drumming are fundamentally different from troupes that do not have a martial arts base. For example, I observed Hong Luck students being sent back for remedial training in kung fu as the antidote to deficiencies in dance skill and musicianship. Given that not all lion dance groups are part of kung fu clubs, context is an important factor in determining whether gong and drum rhythms are acting as martial sound. I am biased towards thinking about martial sound as an integral component of some Southern Chinese kung fu styles because of the ways that transmission, practice, and performance established discourses that constructed it that way during my fieldwork. My consultants explicitly accorded rhythm a place in both fighting applications and choreographed martial arts performance, although the finesse of their physical demonstrations belied their limited verbalization of the matter. This ethnography of Hong Luck's practices treats kung fu, lion dance, and percussion as inseparable components of their Southern Chinese martial arts as a blurred genre.

Embodied Knowing in a Kung Fu Stance

In 1985, Joseph Kerman's book *Contemplating Music* announced the beginnings of a New Musicology. He called for a type of music criticism informed by ethnomusicology and its humanities-oriented approach, which would mark a break from positivism and pure musical analysis. Kerman self-consciously pointed out that the study of music tends to lag behind other academic disciplines in terms of its acceptance of general intellectual trends and that "semiotics, hermeneutics, and phenomenology are being drawn upon only by some of the boldest of musical studies today" (1985: 17). Since then, music scholars have gone considerably further in their theoretical engagement. The following summary of these developments is intended to be brief enough that the review will not be overly tiresome for my fellow ethnomusicologists, but it also needs to provide sufficient detail to orient an interdisciplinary audience. Moreover, some traditionalists continue to challenge the use of such theories and methods in music scholarship, and so I am setting up a proleptic adjustment to pre-defend my choices from criticism.

In the seminal edited volume on ethnomusicological fieldwork *Shadows in the Field* (ed. Barz and Cooley 2008 [1997]), Harris Berger, Timothy Rice, and Jeff Titon all contributed articles arguing for the value of phenomenology in music ethnography. The origins of this continental European philosophical tradition lie in the work of the German philosopher Edmund Husserl (1859–1938) and his slogan "to the 'things themselves'" (1970 [1900]: 252). Husserl's key insight was that consciousness is always consciousness of something, and he laid out the horizons of experience as the essential ground for research into phenomena (1962 [1913]: 223). More specifically, experiences are intentional because people must focus on specific aspects of their existence; if phenomena had no foreground and background through intentionality, the cognitive noise would be overwhelming. By turning towards the intentionality of consciousness, subject and object are linked together, although Husserl also called for intersubjective verification to rule out solipsism, insanity, hallucinations, or dreams. Phenomenology is integral to my work because much of my research hinges on investigating my own embodied experiences as a member of Hong Luck and the way those experiences have been consciously shaped by the club's teachers, seniors, and elders.

Martin Heidegger, one of Husserl's students, developed a style of existential phenomenology that was influenced by Daoism (May 1996 [1989]; ed.

Parkes 1987) and has resonances with kung fu's ethos. Briefly, Daoism is a Chinese philosophy referred to as Teachings of the Way [*Douh Gaau*, 道教], where the Way or Dao [*Douh*, 道] is the supreme principle of the universe with which practitioners seek to align themselves. In Heidegger's essay on artwork, artist, and art (1977 [1950]), he argued for a recursive ontology where the artist creates the artwork and the artwork creates the artist. For Heidegger, art exists to un-conceal a world, and its work is to guide people into an authentic way of being-in-the-world. Artist, artwork, and audience must all participate together in this worlding. For Heidegger, the Being of beings is always "there-being" (*Da-sein*), and, as with Husserl, being-in-the-world is thus contingent on subjects' relationships to the objects of their reality. Southern Chinese kung fu has a strong influence from Daoism and parallels Heidegger's description of visual arts; martial artists use movement and sound to perform martial arts, and martial arts training creates martial artists. Phenomenologically speaking, kung fu training provides a way of being-in-the-world, which allows martial arts to act as modes of revealing being.

Presenting a considerable affinity with the basis of phenomenological thought, Titon has characterized the emergent paradigm of ethnomusicology as the study of "people making and experiencing music" (2008 [1997]: 29). He goes on to suggest that the epistemology of ethnomusicology is fundamentally phenomenological because it is rooted in fieldwork, music, and relationships; what we can know is understood in and as experience (rather than just explained as abstract sound), and we know it by sharing musical being-in-the-world with our consultants. This type of knowledge is emergent, self-reflexive, and contestable, but also grounded by the connections between the people who make and experience any given music (or martial sound). In terms of how to apply the style of phenomenology that Titon advocates, philosopher Don Ihde has suggested that the best method is to acquire the requisite attitude, but not to become mired in jargon (2007 [1976]: 19). In this book, I follow ethnomusicologists like Titon (1988) who exemplify Ihde's approach by their use of a phenomenological attitude towards ethnography, but who do not let their writing get bogged down by philosophical terminology (see also Rice 1994; Stone 1982).

Given the practice-led nature of my research, I also draw on Pierre Bourdieu's practice theory (1977 [1972], 1990 [1980]). I am in good company here, because his conceptual framework has acted as a lens for other ethnographic work in ethnomusicology (e.g., Monson 1999; Rice 1994; Sugarman

1989; Turino 2000), in dance (Cowan 1990; Ness 1992), and in martial arts studies (Downey 20025; Farrer 2009; Lewis 1992; eds. Spencer and García 2013). Bourdieu's influential model is built around *habitus*, which refers to the sets of embodied dispositions that unconsciously structure people's actions. Society conditions these structuring structures over time, and they can be generalized between different aspects of life, leading to embodied practical logic that is both durable and economical. Reifying the habitus or pursuing thinly veiled structuralism is not the point. Instead, practice involves agency though a "generative principle of regulated improvisations" (Bourdieu 1977 [1972]: 78).

In a useful countermeasure to the purported durability of Bourdieu's structuring structures, sociologist Dale Spencer has used a phenomenological approach to discuss the production of a martial artist's habitus "as a lived-through structure-in-process that is continually subject to change through learning additional body techniques" (2009: 120). A Chinese kung fu habitus must thus be considered emergent because it is inculcated through the gradual acquisition of skill in an institutional setting, rather than acquired from familial and communal socialization since birth. The rigorous physical regimen of martial arts practice instils transferable schemata that are at once bodily and socio-cultural. Inasmuch as the habitus is both producer and product of these martial practices, it inhabits the intersection of self and other through teaching, learning, training, and applying. Just as there is no end to kung fu, so practitioners' habitus must be considered a perpetual work-in-progress.

Phenomenological concern for lived experience and sociological interest in structuring structures have a point of intersection in the interpretation of expressive culture. In order to draw together these two streams of theory, I will deploy Harris Berger's (2009) concept called *stance*. He defines it as "the affective, stylistic, or valual quality with which a person engages with an element of her experience" (2009: xiv). Berger proposes that the constitution of lived meaning can be studied by attending to the culturally specific ways in which people engage with experience and that those structures are a type of social practice. From a stance perspective, the formal properties of music, dance, drama, martial arts, or any other type of expressive culture are not simply repositories of meaning whose "text" is interpreted according to the context of society and history. Instead, the structures of experience emerge through a dialectic between agency and culture. Meaning is actively constituted as performers and audiences grapple with the qualities of present-experience in relation to the sediment of past-experience. Social norms and cultural models guide what and how people express, but do not pre-determine the process. The qualia of people's stances arise as their culturally conditioned abilities guide the intentionality of their consciousness; practical logic both enables and constrains their agentive action towards phenomena. Berger's stance theory provides a model for engaging with the dynamics of emergent meanings by showing how text and context are both experienced as aspects of practice.

The idea of stance is not only a helpful way of combining phenomenology and practice theory, but also an *apropos* fit for discussing kung fu. In many styles of Chinese martial arts, including Hong Luck's, the fundamental pose is a deep squat with the feet set wide apart and the torso held vertically, which looks as though one is riding an invisible horse. The "horse stance" [*sei pìhng máah*, 四平馬] is the default posture for kung fu, lion dance, and drumming. At Hong Luck, horse-stance training is fundamental because it builds both physical strength and self-discipline. Beginners practise the position every class by holding it for extended periods of time; they must develop the ability to stay low even as their legs burn and shake from exertion. As I will explain in Chapter 3, it would be hard to overestimate the importance of the horse stance in constructing kung fu being-in-the-world. Berger's stance concept fits into this schema by providing a theoretical framework for thinking about how martial arts inculcate dispositions and positionality through physical training in the horse stance, as well as how practitioners and audiences engage with kung fu phenomena through the structures of their past and present experiences. In the same way that the ambiguity of kung fu's meaning as martial arts and/or acquired skill is rich with interpretive potential, so is stance's meaning because it includes both kung fu's fundamental physical position as well as an embodied *stance on* sense and significance.

Apprenticeship as Fieldwork

I joined Hong Luck with the intention of using participant observation as my primary fieldwork method for studying their drumming, and my consultants guided me towards a culturally appropriate way of applying that approach: apprenticeship. Whereas bi-musicality (Hood 1960) has long been important in ethnomusicology, my apprenticeship also required extensive physical training to acquire not only musical ability but also cultural proficiency in bodily arts. It also encouraged my fieldwork consultants to collaborate in my research by shaping my emerging skills in ways that were familiar to them and that reflected their concerns, values, and beliefs. Apprenticeship as method means undergoing a socially conditioned transformation from novice towards practitioner whereby tradition-bearers use their established transmission process to impart embodied knowledge, to discipline variation, and ultimately shape the body-mind of the researcher (Downey, Dalidowicz, and Mason 2014). The process at Hong Luck was iterative and recursive, moving from demonstration to imitation, repetition, correction, improvement, and back to re-demonstration. In terms of what I studied, "apprenticeship is not only an excellent way to learn a skill; it is also an ideal way to *learn about* it, and to *learn about how one learns*" (italics in original, Downey, Dalidowicz, and Mason 2014: 3). In line with kung fu's literal meaning, being an apprentice revealed the ways in which one achieves skill through effort over time, as well as how that process determines what one knows about it. Put another way, "technique is knowledge that structures practice" (Spatz 2015: 10); apprenticeship uses enskillment to build knowing.

Apprenticeship benefits from careful attention to the corporeal dimensions of experience and existence, and it is a process measured in years, not months. Hong Luck's required progression from martial arts, to lion dance, and finally percussion necessitated a long-term commitment. In contrast to ethnographers who must travel great distances to reach their fieldwork sites, I had the luxury of living near to Hong Luck. Without this proximity, it would have been impossible for me to learn to drum according to their traditional transmission process. Another kung fu club might have been willing to let me learn their drumming separately from martial arts and lion dance, or let me use expedient means that differed from their customary pedagogy, either of which would have changed the nature of my project. Along those lines, Michael Bakan (1999) negotiated the use of Western music notation in his gamelan drumming lessons in Bali to accelerate his learning and fit into the time limits of his fieldwork period. Although his method differed significantly from the traditional way of learning, Bakan argued that his pragmatic goal was being able to play music with local musicians in an acceptable way as quickly as possible. He argued that using any means necessary would allow him to focus on investigating the shared intercultural exchange, as opposed to a more typically bi-musical approach to understanding the music "from within." While that method worked for Bakan's situation and objectives, painstaking apprenticeship at Hong Luck has revealed a world that would not have been available to me if I had focused on learning drumming alone. The challenges of approaching martial sound through kung fu and lion dance meant not only copious amounts of sweat and sore muscles, but also sprains, strains, scrapes, cuts, blisters, and bruises, not to mention one particularly bloody nose and a couple of broken ribs. It was not easy, but, despite the rigours of the transmission process, it was actually a lot of fun.

The requisite kung fu training that I undertook parallels the "carnal" research method espoused by sociologist Loïc Wacquant (2004) in his groundbreaking work at an inner-city boxing club in Chicago. As fieldwork, he trained assiduously there for three and a half years, culminating in a pugilistic baptism by fire when he fought in a Golden Gloves boxing match. Through incorporating the concept of habitus into hands-on research, Wacquant writes that his study of an African American boxing gym "is better characterized as an 'observant participation'" (2004: 6). By inverting the well-known *participant-observation* method to become *observant participation*, Wacquant is recognizing that this type of fieldwork immerses the ethnographer and precludes any illusion of "objective" observation. He acknowledges that fieldwork on—and with—the body has elements of auto-ethnography, but he balances this in his study by documenting both the physical process of his boxer's apprenticeship and also the inseparably social aspects.

Ethnicity can intersect apprenticeship, which speaks to how Wacquant-style embodied research raises issues of race and culture in regard to habitus. For example, in their research on Brazilian capoeira in Britain, sociologists Sara Delamont and Neil Stephens (2008) interrogate the discourses of identity that are confronted by non-Brazilian *capoeiristas* (as adepts are called). As I have already explained, many aspects of a person's habitus are formed early in life, perhaps definitively so in conservative mono-cultural societies, but other elements may be acquired later. Delamont and Stephens use practice theory to investigate adults building the habits and dispositions of capoeira in a diasporic context, focusing on the way British students negotiate Brazilian culture through enskillment. Researching Chinese kung fu in multicultural Toronto raised a similar issue, where the Chinese-ness of kung fu was often emphasized, despite Hong Luck's Canadian location and multiethnic membership. As a European Canadian performing ethnography in a diasporic Chinese martial arts club, my white skin made my Caucasian ethnicity impossible to mistake. Nonetheless, Hong Luck members explicitly maintained that practising kung fu can make any body more Chinese (even mine), which suggests their awareness of how movement and sound can affect a person's habitus.

By blurring the boundaries between researcher and research subject, my work is also a form of performance ethnography. As such, I have found it necessary to sometimes switch my writing voice between that of a scholar and that of a performer. Deborah Wong (2008 [1997]) discusses this sort of performative ethnography in her research on *taiko* drumming from her perspective as a *taiko* drummer. Performance ethnography of the sort I undertook at Hong Luck also benefits from theory that explicitly addresses how one might bridge the emic/etic divide. Timothy Rice's solution is to use Ricoeur's hermeneutic arc to recursively connect insider and outsider perspectives in order to achieve an understanding that can contribute novel insights (1994: 72). Through his personal struggles to learn the ornamentation required to play the Bulgarian bagpipes (*gaida*) in a culturally acceptable way, Rice posits a subject position for ethnomusicological researchers that balances personal lived experience and acquired knowledge in a dynamic interpretation. In a similar vein, Michael Bakan defends his focus on his own experience of learning to play the drum used in Balinese gamelan *beleganjur* by arguing, "[t]he ways we construct, contest, and experience our worlds determine what we understand and how we understand" (1999: 331). Since the self-reflexive and interpretative turn of the social sciences and humanities in the 1980s, a view like Bakan's has become more common, but its ramifications bear repeating: addressing the ethnographer's experience as a valid phenomenon for research does not suggest that it is the same as that of the informant, but rather that both are part of the shared world that arises during fieldwork.

Altogether, it took approximately five years before I could play the drum for performances in an acceptable style, although I stayed at Hong Luck for a further three years to refine my skills and knowledge, and I only left the club when I moved to Ireland to take up the fellowship that funded me to write this book. Part of why I remained after completing my primary fieldwork was in deference to what I perceived as a debt to the club, its members, and their traditions. I continued to volunteer as a lion dancer and drummer to help raise money for Hong Luck, which is a registered not-for-profit organization in the Province of Ontario. I also helped teach kung fu, lion dance, and percussion to pass on some of the knowledge that I had received. While this book is an academic monograph that documents, analyzes, and interprets my fieldwork data, it is perhaps more importantly an extension of my commitment to Hong Luck's mandate of preserving and promoting kung fu.

Ethnography and Propriety

During eight years of fieldwork, Hong Luck members shared a vast amount of insider knowledge with me, some of which I am not at liberty to share with outsiders. While not themselves prone to quoting Confucius, my consultants guided me towards maintaining "propriety" [fānchyun, 分寸], which is an important Confucian value that aims to align speech and behaviour with social norms. My fieldwork situation raised some issues of research propriety, which are not unlike those that James Kippen (2008 [1997]) experienced as a disciple studying tablā drumming in northern India. Kippen reflects on occasional friction between disciplinary loyalty to accurate ethnomusicological scholarship and discipular loyalty to his ustād (master musician and guru) whose information could at times be fictive or instrumental. Doing research at Hong Luck meant working both to develop my kung fu in the broadest sense of the word and to fit into the "martial forest" [móuhlàhm, 武林], as the life-world of kung fu practitioners is sometimes known. Earning a place within the social order of Hong Luck's pseudo-kinship structure allowed me to be privy to their martial sound, including aspects that are not usually performed in public. Out of respect for my consultants, I have adapted my research outputs to maintain propriety in three areas: confidentiality, hierarchy, and notation.

Three months into my fieldwork, I was invited to join the lion dance class. I dutifully informed the teacher of my research activities, whereupon he laid down ground rules. His first rule had to do with protecting people's privacy, which is common practice in ethnographic research anyway. I keep the contributions of Hong Luck members pseudonymous, anonymous, or recognized by name according to their wishes and my view of best practice. For example, my first lion dance teacher wished to keep his participation in kung fu private, and so I have removed identifying personal details and shall refer to him by the pseudonym Noah throughout this book. On the other hand, my second lion dance teacher, and main drumming mentor, wished to be recognized for his contributions to my research and so I use his real name, David Lieu (Láuh Gā-wáih, 柳嘉偉). For people who had less sustained input, it is more expedient to refer to them in generally anonymous ways.

For figures like Master Paul Chan and Master Jim Chan, who were publicly known as martial artists during their lives and have now passed on, I use their real names out of respect.

Some members wished to be anonymous because they were being modest, which is a valued trait in Chinese culture, but others were being careful. As one member explained to me, if people know that one does martial arts, it can result in challenges to fight. Furthermore, one loses the advantage of a secret weapon if an assailant is aware that one knows kung fu. As an example of this type of secrecy, one senior member told me she refers to Hong Luck as "KFC" (an acronym for kung fu club) because outsiders would think she was talking about the fast-food restaurant historically known as Kentucky Fried Chicken. For similar reasons, I have omitted information on historical connections between Hong Luck and Chinese secret societies.

The second ground rule came in the form of learning to respect my place in the club's social and pedagogical hierarchy. Noah told me that the founding elders of Hong Luck were off-limits to me for interview requests; they would decide if/when they would engage with me. Some of these men were still active around the club, but they typically chose to be involved only with the more advanced students. Noah said that being a researcher did not give me special privileges in that regard, and so I would need to advance my position before earning the attention of the club's elders. I eventually had conversations or lessons with these elders, but it occurred through accepted martial or social paths, rather than as researcher-directed contact. As my skills improved, for example, Master Paul Chan noticed me and began to offer occasional tips on lion dance and kung fu. In 2014, a senior instructor invited me to join Master Jim Chan's advanced class, where I received regular lessons on kung fu and somewhat less frequent coaching on the drum. I also had the good fortune of sitting with several elders at communal tables during meals, as well as in the training hall after classes at Hong Luck, which allowed me to engage them in informal chat. In some ways, the delay in getting access to Hong Luck elders was good, because by the time I got to speak with them more regularly, my ongoing efforts to learn Cantonese were paying off. Hong Luck's two founding masters were native Taishanese speakers who could speak Cantonese as a second language, but they had limited English. My language abilities proved particularly useful when I joined Master Jim Chan's class, as he was clearly more comfortable in Chinese and usually spoke a mix of Cantonese and Taishanese with a few English words or phrases for emphasis.

Kung fu skills accrue gradually, so eager students—and researchers—must develop their patience lest they be accused of trying to "steal learning" [*tāu hohk*, 偷學]. Towards the end of my first year of fieldwork, Noah agreed to do a recorded ethnographic interview with me, but it proved minimally productive. As Jonathan Stock has noted (2004), long-term participant-observation sometimes provide far more data than direct questions. Asking my teachers or the elders either specific or broad questions about martial arts, lion dance, or drumming might have gotten me answers, but they were never complete. I thus only did a handful of formal interviews where I either recorded audio or took notes. These were helpful for clarifying factual details or confirming theories, but they yielded relatively little new information or direct quotes. In many cases, Hong Luck members showed me the things they wanted me to know, rather than told me about them.

Because of the way my fieldwork progressed, the text of this book bears few direct quotations. Instead, I often rely on paraphrases or summaries of ongoing conversations that may have been spread out over months or even years. Occasionally, my consultants have had concise-but-deep things to say that stuck in my memory, or they have repeated certain things often enough to drill them into me. I will cite such examples word for word. After years of not only apprenticing but also performing and socializing with Hong Luck members, my work resembles what Jeff Titon (2008 [1997]: 37–40) has called a *friendship model*. I got to know my classmates and teachers in situ, which brought their views, beliefs, and concerns to the fore over time. Casual conversation ended up being a good source of information, so it is fortunate that there were many opportunities for indirect and informal interaction as part of what Clifford Geertz (1998) calls *deep hanging out*. After lion dance gigs, for example, the group usually had dinner together, and there were also yearly anniversary banquets involving Hong Luck's full membership. Before and after training sessions, there were plenty of chances to chat, too, so I often turned the conversation towards topics pertinent to my research, but it was typically in a dialogical mode, rather than an investigative one.

The third rule that Noah laid down was not to write out the percussion rhythms in Western staff notation—at least not until I could play them from memory to his satisfaction.[5] It was not that he prevented students from documenting the rhythms entirely (audiovisual recording was deemed

---

[5] While there were no prohibitions against writing field notes, this was not practical during sweat-drenched classes or performances, and so it had to wait until I got home.

acceptable); rather my teacher was concerned that I should come to understand the beats through the customary transmission process. He told me that if I just transcribed the rhythms, I might miss what was important about them regarding embodied knowledge of lion dance and kung fu. When David took over the lion dance class from Noah, he escalated the prohibition of music notation, arguing that the rhythms should never be written down at all. Several other senior members, however, argued that it would be good for me to transcribe as much of the club's rhythmic repertoire as possible in order to preserve it for Hong Luck's private archive, although they did not want those transcriptions published. David still felt that the substitution of visual, two-dimensional notation was insufficient to represent the phenomenon, but paradoxically it could also potentially leak secrets that people had not earned. David believed that notation could allow people—Hong Luck members or otherwise—to learn the drum rhythms the "wrong" way. The correct method of transmission was aural, oral, physical, and person-to-person. Notwithstanding the differences of opinion among Hong Luck members about music notation, I deferred to David's wishes because he became my main drumming mentor.

During the fall and winter terms of 2011/2012, I went on an academic exchange to the Chinese University of Hong Kong [*Jūngmàhn Daaihhohk*, 中文大學] to study Cantonese, as well as get more familiar with lion dance and kung fu in Greater China. While I was there, I found Chinese-language texts that contained transcriptions of skeletal or normative versions of the lion dance rhythms, which I copied and brought home (eds. Li and Liu 1985; Liang 2008). David was interested to see these and softened his position somewhat by allowing me to do some transcription to facilitate communicating my research. He remained firm, however, in his opposition to providing longer transcriptions or exhaustive documentation of motivic variations. This is not to say that he did not support my research, but rather that he was more comfortable with me analysing, explaining, and interpreting phenomena that would help my readers understand these practices, without giving away certain types of detail. Consistent with Hong Luck's overall transmission process, he prioritized embodied knowledge and lived experience.

There were also limits placed on my ability to share audiovisual material. Although my active participation precluded me from recording many videos myself, club members often filmed their own recordings, which they were kind enough to share with me. I also eventually got access to archival videos from performances dating back as far as thirty years. Hong Luck members circulated these recordings via burned DVDs, but the older recordings had been transferred from video cassettes. When I received copies from people, they typically warned me not to share them with outsiders and especially not to post them online. Towards the end of my fieldwork at Hong Luck, however, discussions among senior members about how to promote the club for lion dance gigs and how to attract more students led to a reconsideration regarding these archival films. After some debate, it was agreed that the benefits of a greater online presence would outweigh the risks of people stealing learning. Volunteers have since posted many video clips online, which can be viewed on Hong Luck's YouTube channel.

Writing Strategies and Plan of Attack

In technical terms, the unfolding of this book parallels the way I learned kung fu, lion dance, and percussion: details are added gradually as I return to the same things from new angles. When dealing with the intersection of such a diverse range of practices, neither a linear progression nor a chronology is really feasible. Kung fu and lion dance form a path for learning how to drum, but that road is rarely straight. As my teachers at Hong Luck did, I have often found myself needing to repeat things to add another layer of detail, meaning, or interpretation that would not have made sense if I had tried to lay it all out the first time I mentioned it. I draw readers' attention to this writing strategy so that necessary repetitions will be taken as recapitulations, rather than duplications.

The plan of this book cycles through the generalities of history, to the specifics of practice, and moves towards the subjectivities of experience. This gradually tightening focus is designed to put context, description, and explanation first in a way that will prevent the book from centering on autoethnography, or worse, devolving into the dreaded "confessional" style. Following the present introduction, the second chapter surveys the origins of Southern Chinese martial arts and lion dance, but it does so in a way that seeks to balance the facts of social history against the equally important place of myths and stories in identity formation. I also outline Chinese experiences in Canada and how a legacy of systemic racism has impacted Chinatown society. The third chapter looks at Hong Luck's main public activity: lion dance. I approach it by detailing symbolic, ritual, cultural, and entertainment perspectives while acknowledging that those lines are blurred in practice. I also explore issues of identity that include negotiation of lion dance protocol, maintaining Hong Luck's distinctive drumming style, and the sonic (re)construction of Chinatown.

The fourth chapter leaves the broad strokes of history and public lion dancing behind to narrow the focus to day-to-day happenings inside the club. Teaching, learning, and practising take up a far greater amount of time than performing or fighting, and it is through training that a kung fu habitus is forged. There I detail physical practice, which Hong Luck explicitly recognizes as embodied cultural education. In the cases of both Canadian-born Chinese and non-Chinese alike, kung fu practice is often a case of acculturation, rather than enculturation. Hong Luck is dedicated to preserving traditional Chinese culture, but members also show their awareness of the complexity and hybridity of a multicultural and multigenerational group of people engaging in these practices in a diasporic context. The through-line of this chapter is the process of developing a Chinese martial arts habitus as the pathway to being able to learn drumming. An important aspect of this route is the network of social relations that constitute the club and give a prospective drummer access to the collective resources of the membership. I also engage with the unmarked masculinity of kung fu. Traditionally, women were excluded from lion dance, which is at odds with Hong Luck's inclusive mandate but speaks to issues of gender in practice and performance.

The fifth and sixth chapters delve into my interpretation of the experience of Hong Luck's martial sound. The hermeneutic will proceed from my own encounter with the percussion and build up to longer ethnographic vignettes of what it is like to demonstrate kung fu, dance under a lion-head mask, and play the big drum that drives performances. An important goal of this book is to further the ability of people outside the (sub)culture to interpret its martial sound by explaining how practitioners and aficionados are experiencing what they hear. I use a cognitive metaphor of synchronization between two vibrating systems to suggest a schema for meaning in Hong Luck's beats. The idea of *entrainment*, as this phenomenon is known, draws on fundamental corporeal knowledge that is available to practitioners and non-practitioners alike in order to discuss choreomusical relationships from a martial perspective. I use this schema to provide an analysis of the rhythm of combat, which builds on my previous work (McGuire 2010, 2015), but takes the discussion further by connecting it to a broader range of practices and contexts.

The last chapter will tie together the different strands of rhythm, movement, and meaning at Hong Luck in order to reflect on the club's legacy. With the deaths of the two founding masters in 2012 and 2016, a new era has begun. One of the key issues facing the next generation of leaders is the preservation of tradition versus the need to reflect a changing world, the negotiation of which is ongoing. Hong Luck continues to be an important part of Toronto's Chinatown community and to act as a bridge with people of other ethnicities. After more than a half century of activity, the club's kung fu and lion dance have left an indelible mark on the physical culture of the Great Toronto Area and beyond, so regardless of the club's future, its impact will continue for years to come. The heroic ideals of self-strengthening and respect for tradition resonate deeply through anyone who identifies with Hong Luck's kung fu, lion dance, and percussion.

2

Histories and Stories

Layered Symbols and Historical Myths

At the back of the Hong Luck Kung Fu Club's training hall, a three-foot statue of an ancient Chinese warrior sits on a throne. Incense smoke and shadows perpetually cloak him in mystery. He is wearing battlefield armour, with one hand raised in an arcane gesture. The altar where he presides has a green tiled roof and raises him up off the floor on a dais, allowing him to gaze down at the training floor from between furrowed brows. Painted on the wall behind him is a coiling dragon, at his feet are ancestral tablets honouring kung fu masters of yore, and on the table in front of him are an array of offerings that include incense braziers, cups of liquor, coins, and fruit. Already ruddy, his face is further incarnadined by a red lightbulb above him, two red electric candles at his feet, and two red lanterns hanging from the ceiling to either side of him. These lights are always on—even at night.

The warrior statue represents Guan Yu [*Gwāan Yú*, 關羽], who is an important figure in Chinese culture and is sometimes known by the exalted title Emperor Guan [*Gwāan Dai*, 關帝].[1] At Hong Luck, he is referred to as General Guan in English or in Cantonese as *Gwāan Gūng* [關公], meaning either *Lord* Guan or *Grandfather* Guan, depending on who you ask and what meaning they derive from the characters in his name.[2] There are Buddhist, Taoist, Confucian, and folk temples devoted to him throughout the Sinophone world, while personal altars to Guan Yu can be found in homes and businesses alike. Diverse groups of people worship him, from elites to common folk, and from police to gangsters. Guan Yu has appeared not only in religion, but also in folk tales, Chinese opera, literature, film, television, advertising, and video games.

---

[1] Guan Yu's name is unsystematically romanized in English, but the most common spelling derives from Mandarin pinyin [*Guān Yǔ*]. The pronunciation of his name is similar in Cantonese. Alternate romanizations of his family name include: Kwan, Gwan, and Kuan.

[2] The ambiguity may stem from the character *gūng* being found in both the compound for "lord duke" [*gūngjeuk*, 公爵] and "paternal grandfather" [*gūnggūng*, 公公].

Martial Sound. Colin P. McGuire, Oxford University Press. © Oxford University Press 2024.
DOI: 10.1093/oso/9780197775936.003.0002

The historical Guan Yu (c.162–220 CE) was an army general; his godly stature in Chinese culture is an apotheosis. He fought in the violent struggles at the close of the Han Dynasty (206 BCE–220 CE). His most famous exploits, however, are as a semi-fictional protagonist in the fourteenth-century novel *Romance of the Three Kingdoms* [*Sāam Gwok Yínyih*, 三國演義]. Over time, a variety of meanings have embroidered Guan Yu's persona, but the main qualities that undergird his cult are bravery, righteousness, and loyalty. He is a god of war, protection, honour, wealth, steadfastness, and allegiance— though not necessarily all at the same time. Practice has deified Guan Yu through discontinuous alternate meanings that remain attached to a continuous core, which historian Prasenjit Duara calls the *superscription of symbols* (1988). According to Duara's concept, Guan Yu is a semiotic palimpsest, such that the inscription of new symbolic value still draws on the power of older myths. As an example of this semantic chaining, some businesspeople worship Guan Yu as a god of wealth, which builds the idea of prosperity on a foundation of protection from loss. At its core, the warrior ethos of a historical army general empowers all imaginings of this important figure.

The importance of Guan Yu to Chinese culture in general, and Hong Luck in particular, makes him a useful metaphor for Chinese martial arts. The idea of symbolic superscription that he embodies acts as a framework for my historical discussion of kung fu, lion dance, and percussion music in this chapter. As Scott Park Phillips (2016) has argued, the fighting pedigree of Chinese martial arts intertwines with music, dance, drama, ritual, religion, and folklore, creating practices that are multivalent in their significance. Each successive layer of meaning in a superscibed sign allows a wider variation of interpretation. As Guan Yu has many aspects, so does kung fu. Contemporary stances on Chinese martial arts, lion dance, and percussion thus draw from multivalent meanings, which people experience in unique ways through a common core.

In this chapter, I engage with the histories and stories that undergird martial sound in Cantonese kung fu. I begin with an overview of Chinese experiences in Canada as context for the formation of Chinatowns and the eventual founding of the Hong Luck Kung Fu Club in 1961. Next, I circle backwards to describe the origins of the kung fu styles practised by my research consultants, which emerged as invented traditions in the mid-nineteenth and early twentieth centuries. Then I explain the roots and symbolism of lion dancing, circling back to martial arts by examining the intersections of lion dance and percussion with Southern Chinese kung fu systems. In keeping with my theory that Hong Luck's kung fu is a blurred genre, I am interested in parsing the amalgamation of combat, ritual, and performance (Jones 2002a), without fully separating them. My point of entry into this area of research is musicking, which is a fully integrated component of the holistic field of practice.

In order to chronicle Hong Luck's lineage, I borrow an approach from subaltern historian Dipesh Chakrabarty (2000). He proposes that inclusive historiography should balance documented facts with the power of stories. Chakrabarty argues that these two things are not antithetical to each other if one treats myth and legend as legitimate sources of influence on people's lives. Stories shape people's life-worlds. Supernatural forces are real when people experience them as agents capable of affecting their lives. Phenomenologically speaking, people take stances on gods, ghosts, demons, angels, and other ethereal energies as actually existing—despite science being incapable of measuring or quantifying them. In a move that brings together an anthropological concern for people's beliefs with a scientific demand for facts, Chakrabarty insists that myths are alternative realities that exist alongside chronological history. He builds this idea on a postcolonial critique of the intellectual violence perpetrated by imposing secular Western historicism onto other peoples. Theoretically, then, paradoxes between histories and stories do not require resolution if one can hold them together in a dynamic interpretation.

Chinese Experiences in Canada

To understand the contemporary context of Hong Luck's martial sound, it is necessary to cover some underexamined history. There have been Chinese people in what is now Canada since before the nation's confederation in 1867, and their experiences have often been difficult. British settlers were both more numerous and politically dominant; for many years, they treated migrants from China as a source of cheap labour—not as potential citizens—forming a pattern that lasted until the middle of the twentieth century (Li 1998: 30). Chinese people made significant contributions to Canadian nation-building through their work on the western portion of the trans-continental railroad. Nonetheless, federal and provincial governments passed numerous laws limiting Chinese immigration, as well as restricting the rights and freedoms of Chinese Canadians. A combination of institutional racism and social discrimination has had a lasting influence on Chinese communities across Canada.

Early Chinese arrivals in Canada came over as labourers. In 1788, British sea-captain John Meares brought the first crew over from China's Guangdong Province to build ships and to construct a fur-trading outpost on the west coast of British Columbia (BC). After a battle with Spanish naval forces in 1789, most of these Chinese carpenters and smiths were killed or captured. According to historian David Lai (2011), some of them likely escaped, but the next extant record of Chinese people in Canada is not until the gold rush along BC's Fraser River in 1858. As with earlier gold rushes in California, recruiters sought Chinese men to work as "coolies"[3] in the mining industry, though others also came independently. Some resentment towards Chinese people was a result of competition for jobs; labourers of European ethnicity commanded higher salaries, and they felt that Chinese workers were undercutting them. Even during labour shortages, however, anti-Chinese sentiment in BC was strong. It drew on legacies of colonialism to construct Chinese people as not only inassimilable, but also as culturally and racially inferior (Li 1998: 31). Gold deposits began to run out in the mid 1860s, diminishing the amount of work for labourers and fuelling discrimination against migrants from China as their perceived "usefulness" decreased.

In 1867, most of the colonies in British North America confederated as the Dominion of Canada, and BC joined in 1871 on the condition that a railway be built to connect the vast resources of the West with the more populated centres of the East, creating renewed demand for cheap labour. Even as Chinese workers already in Canada found jobs laying railroad tracks and new recruits arrived from Guangdong Province, the government was passing legislation against them. By the early 1870s, physical segregation laws in the BC cities of Victoria, Nanaimo, and Kamloops resulted in the formation of Canada's first Chinese-only neighbourhoods, a.k.a. Chinatowns (Lai 2011). Later came disenfranchisement of Chinese people by the province of BC in 1875 (Li 1998: 32). Furthermore, by preventing labourers from bringing their wives or children with them, Canadian authorities hoped that Chinese sojourners would return home after finishing their projects.

The completion of the transcontinental railway in 1885 meant there was no longer an urgent need for cheap labour, and the situation became direr.

---

[3] The word *coolie* comes from the Mandarin term *kǔlì*, meaning "bitter toil" [Cantonese: *fúlihk*, 苦力].

Many Chinese already in Canada began moving east looking for work, while administrative wheels turned to oppress them and stop their population from increasing. In order to prevent more Chinese from coming to Canada, the federal government passed laws restricting their immigration, notably in the form of a so-called Head Tax that was not applicable to other ethnic or national groups. The Head Tax was apparently ineffective because the Chinese population nearly doubled in the decade between 1891 and 1901, going from 9,129 to 17,312 (Li 1998: 89). The levy started at $50 for each immigrant from China, was raised to $100 in 1900, and reached $500 in 1903. At the same time, various other provincial and federal laws limited what occupations migrants from China could hold. Although Chinese people were not barred from post-secondary education, they were not allowed to enter professions like law or medicine. This process culminated in the Chinese Immigration Act (a.k.a. the Chinese Exclusion Act) of 1923 that slowed immigration to a trickle until its repeal in 1947.

As a result of the various pressures I have just outlined, the vast majority of Chinese Canadians were, for many years, concentrated in Chinatowns and had distinctive social structures. They were mostly male, spoke little English, and worked in an ethnic economy consisting of the few industries available to them: restaurants, groceries, laundries, and garment manufacturing. With limited access to banking, police, education, politics, or government services, they relied on a network of benevolent fraternal associations to fill the gap. On the one hand, discrimination forced these men into Chinatowns. On the other, their stance on their neighbourhood was one of familiarity, comfort, and support thanks to the mutual-aid groups. Chinatown benevolent associations are sometimes known as "tongs" [tòhng, 堂], referring to a meeting hall. They have often functioned as secret societies whose activities are open only to members. The tong system remains active in Canada and the United States, although these groups are no longer as pervasive or as powerful as they once were. The Hong Luck Kung Fu Club is one type of tong.

For many years, fraternal tong societies formed the centre of social, economic, and political life in Chinatown. They were based on a kinship model, so people with the same family name would belong to a common clan association, such as Chan [Chàhn, 陳] or Lee [Léih, 李]. There were also place-based associations for people from the same counties in China's Guangdong Province, such as Taishan. Finally, there were associations like Hong Luck that functioned as a catch-all for people of different backgrounds, although their hierarchies still followed a vertical kinship structure rooted in Confucian values of filial piety, respect for elders, and group loyalty. Throughout the Chinese diaspora, tong associations embraced a multitude of functions. Anthropologist Richard H. Thompson has summarized the roles of these societies in Toronto thusly:

> (1) ritual—the organization and celebration of traditional Chinese festivals such as New Year, the Ching Ming festival, the Mid-Autumn festival; (2) social—ownership of a house or hall which served as a center for conversation, gambling, games, and for a few individuals, a rooming house; (3) social-welfare—this included caring for the sick, arranging for the burial of deceased members; (4) economic—providing job placement and operating rotating credit associations known as *hui*; (5) political—settling disputes between members, sanctioning their behaviour, and representing them in their infrequent contacts with Canadian authorities. (1989: 75)

In the case of Hong Luck, kung fu club and tong association are related but distinct, sharing the same three-story building but also remaining somewhat separate. During my fieldwork, members referred to the tong branch of the group as Hong Luck Upstairs because martial arts practice occurred on the main floor (with change rooms in the basement), while the association's other activities happened on the second and third floors. Martial artists were not automatically part of the Hong Luck tong association, however, and there were also association members who did not practise martial arts. Hong Luck Upstairs provided stewardship and financial backing for the kung fu club, which was a registered with the Province of Ontario as a not-for-profit organization. Most of the senior members of the kung fu branch (i.e., my primary fieldwork consultants) were part of both divisions, and eventually they invited me to become a part of Hong Luck Upstairs, too. They requested that I limit the amount of detail—past or present—that I provide about Hong Luck's non–kung fu activities. The secretive world of the tongs reflects the social and institutional marginalization that Chinese Canadians faced. Hong Luck members taking such a stance on privacy therefor came as no surprise.

A key factor in the success of the tong network was the relative cultural and linguistic homogeneity of Chinese communities in Canada before 1970. Most early Chinese migrants in Canada were from what are colloquially known in Cantonese as the *Sei Yāp* [four counties, 四邑] and *Sāam Yāp* [three counties, 三邑] regions of Guangdong province. In Toronto, a large majority of the Chinese population hailed from villages in the Taishan district of the Sei Yap (Thompson 1989: 45–49). The founders of Hong Luck are no exception to this pattern.

The laws of China's Qing Dynasty forbade emigration, but Taishanese men still managed to leave in droves thanks to the position of Taishan on the coast and its proximity to Hong Kong, as well as the connections of Taishanese people to the sea trade (Li 1998: 17–20). Taishan county lies along the mountainous coastline to the southwest of Guangzhou city, the provincial capital of Guangdong Province. The terrain limits arable land, and population growth in the nineteenth century outstripped sustainable agriculture. As a result, many men sought work as intermediaries between arriving ships and the cities of the Pearl River Delta. During that period, unequal treaties with European powers and rebellions in other parts of China created a desperate situation in China that led the men of Taishan to seek their fortunes overseas.

Historian Henry Yu has identified a century-long process of circular migration along oceanic shipping routes, which he calls the Cantonese Pacific (Yu 2013). From the 1850s to the mid-twentieth century, Cantonese migrants established patterns of relocation connecting Guangdong with North America, South East Asia, and Oceania. Some left China never to return, while others finished their sojourns and came back, or sometimes made several trips back and forth. This process established durable, long-distance connections of family, friendship, business, and politics around the Pacific. Hong Kong was the crucial port for international Cantonese departures because of the city's connection to the British Commonwealth and its position on the trade routes of US territories. During this period, there was also significant outwards migration from neighbouring Fujian Province to Southeast Asia, but Hong Kong was the gateway to the larger Cantonese Pacific.

As I have already explained, the original migrants from China came to BC for the gold rush and to build the railroad, but by 1878 the first of them had made his way east (Lai and Leong 2012). Toronto is the capital of Canada's most populous province, Ontario, and not later than 1920, a Chinatown began to form around the current location of Nathan Philips Square in the city's downtown core. Only a few remnants of the early Chinese Canadian neighbourhood remain. When the city of Toronto started building a new municipal complex during the 1960s, it expropriated a large chunk of land, including parts of the original Chinatown. At the same time, investors began buying as much nearby property as they could, which drove real-estate prices up and limited opportunities for new Chinese businesses or homes in the area (Chan 2011). Expropriation and speculation forced the Chinese community to move a few blocks west to its current location around the intersection of Spadina Avenue and Dundas Street West.

In 1967, the Canadian government established a universal point system for immigration, which was a major turning point for the old Chinatown system. While the 1947 repeal of the Chinese Exclusion Act had allowed some immigration from China, the new point system removed the final barriers and allowed the first large-scale influx of Chinese people to Canada since 1923. The twenty-year period between the end of Chinese exclusion in 1947 and the universal point system in 1967 was a time of transition for Chinatown communities in Canada. Demographics gradually transitioned from being primarily adult men to also including their wives and children. Despite the increasing diversity of gender and age, Toronto's Chinese community remained primarily Taishanese-speaking in the inter-years because it was easier for established people to sponsor new immigrants and reunite their families. Under Canada's new point system, however, Cantonese-speaking people from Hong Kong began to dominate Chinese immigration after 1967. As citizens of a British colony, many of them knew some English, which earned them extra credit for their applications. Much of this new wave of immigration was driven by fears surrounding the return of Hong Kong to Chinese rule in 1997. By the 1980s, the majority of Chinese Canadians were still Cantonese in the broad sense, but people from urban Hong Kong eclipsed those from rural Taishan (Li 1998).

As Toronto's Chinese community grew and matured, the tong system persisted, but it also faced different types of pressure. Cultural commonalities in the Chinese Canadian population helped hold the tongs together, while improved circumstances for the community reduced the need for mutual aid. Urban Cantonese and rural Taishanese are partially mutually intelligible, sharing a common root as dialects of Yue Chinese. Furthermore, both come from the Pearl River Delta region of Guangdong Province. Speakers of these dialects thus share many aspects of culture. Nonetheless, there arose class differences in Toronto between the new and old immigrants based on education, language, and the rural/urban divide (Thompson 1989: 23). As one senior Hong Luck member put it, the difference between Taishanese and Hong Kong people was like "country mouse and city mouse," meaning they were all ethnolinguistically Cantonese, but they were divided by subtle differences of language and culture. Newcomers from Hong Kong, as well as the Canadian-born children of the established Chinese community, were more likely to be bilingual in a dialect of Yue Chinese and English. They took advantage of relaxed labour laws and increasing social acceptance of diversity. They also had access to government-funded social services and the Canadian banking system. Class distinctions, combined with increased opportunity resulting from the lessening of institutional discrimination, contributed to a gradual erosion of the traditional tong system's importance.

Established Chinese Canadians gradually dispersed around the Greater Toronto Area, and new immigrants replaced them in Chinatown, resulting in a dilution of the linguistic and cultural homogeneity in the neighbourhood surrounding the Hong Luck Kung Fu Club. Over time, Canada has received waves of Chinese immigrants from several locations in the broader diaspora: Southeast Asia, the Caribbean, and Taiwan. Since emigration regulations in the People's Republic of China (PRC) relaxed in the mid 1980s,[4] there has been a marked increase of immigrants from Chinese provinces other than Guangdong, each with their own native dialect but also speaking Mandarin as a common tongue. When Hong Luck was founded, the lingua franca of Chinatown was rural Taishanese; by the 1980s it had become urban Cantonese, and now there is a rise in the national language of China. The PRC has long promoted Mandarin as its official tongue, so it is not surprising that increasing linguistic diversity in Chinatown has led to an increase in Mandarin usage. Immigration from a wider range of regions in China has also changed what it means to be Chinese in Canada, which has in some ways diminished support for Hong Luck's Cantonese practices.

Today, the established network of benevolent associations still exists in Toronto's Spadina/Dundas Chinatown, but it functions at reduced capacity. Their membership is aging. Canadian-born Chinese appear to have less interest in—or need for—the tongs. At the same time, new mutual-aid groups have arisen that support recent arrivals to Canada and connect them to more established Chinese Canadians. For example, the Taishan Friendship Association of Ontario [*Gānàhdaaih Ōnsáang Tòihsāan Tùhnghēung Lyùhnhahp Júngwúi*, 加拿大安省台山同鄉聯合總會] was founded in 2010 and has a vibrant membership that includes men, women, and children. Their mandate is different than the older tongs, however, and focuses on

---

[4] From its founding in 1949 until the 1980s, the PRC strove to limit the number of people leaving the mainland, thus making Hong Kong the main source of Chinese migration to Canada in the mid-twentieth century. That being said, people from Guangdong were sometimes able to get across the PRC's border to Hong Kong, meaning that Cantonese people had better emigration opportunities than they would have in other parts of the mainland. The processes of the Cantonese Pacific have thus persisted beyond the initial century of migration.

developing social, political, and business interests. This group does not have their own building, but rather the administrators meet at Hong Luck. In fact, many of the Taishan Friendship Association's leaders are members of Hong Luck Upstairs. The growth of this new tong has been a boon for the kung fu club because their patronage of lion dance has injected some much-needed income into the flagging coffers.

History of the Hong Luck Kung Fu Club

As I mentioned in Chapter 1, two Southern Chinese martial arts masters founded Hong Luck in 1961. Despite sharing a surname and both hailing from Taishan county in China, Master Paul Chan and Master Jim Chan first met while working at a restaurant in Toronto's old Chinatown. Master Paul was a natural leader, endowed with an outgoing personality, an imposing physique, and an indomitable fighting spirit. He was the chief instructor and public face of the club from its beginning till his death in 2012. Master Jim had a more reserved character, making important contributions as the vice-principal instructor through his tremendous refinement of kung fu, particularly in regard to martial performance. One long-time Hong Luck member described them as the club's right and left hands, playing different roles that were both essential to the group's success. Nonetheless, Master Paul's long tenure as the chief instructor gives him pride of place in Hong Luck's history.

Together, Masters Paul and Jim formed Hong Luck with eleven other Chinese Canadian men, meeting in several ad hoc locations around old Chinatown throughout the early 1960s. During the exodus to make way for Toronto's new City Hall and Nathan Philips Square, Hong Luck members put together funds to purchase and renovate their own building in new Chinatown. Since 1968, the group's permanent location has been a three-story house located at 548 Dundas Street West.

The club's mandate was spelled out for me by one of the original elders, whom Hong Luck member's referred to (in Cantonese) as "Uncle" Poi [*Pùih Sūk*, 培叔] (pers. Comm, November 24, 2013)[5]:

1. Teach kung fu as a pursuit for healthy body and mind
2. Promote use of kung fu for self-defence only

---

[5] Uncle Poi's full name is Ńgh Jípùih [伍梓培].

3. Promote kung fu as a common interest in the Chinese and broader Canadian communities to come together for learning, greater cultural understanding, and peace
4. Outreach to all associations for the betterment of Canadian society

Uncle Poi used the word *kung fu* in the broad sense I discussed in Chapter 1, referring not only to fighting skills, but also martial performance, lion dance, and percussion. His summary of the club's mandate highlights a central paradox at Hong Luck, which is also found in many other styles of hand combat. Martial arts can be used to resist and embrace, to break and build, to divide and connect. On the one hand, Hong Luck members practised fighting skills to defend themselves against racist aggression. On the other, they used the same fighting skills to make connections with people from outside Chinatown. Whether through teaching or performance, Hong Luck's kung fu has acted as strategic diplomacy, building bridges between the Chinese Canadian community and non–Chinese Canadians. The club's stance on self-defence shows advanced strategic positioning; the best way to win a fight is by not fighting at all.

Because of the changing role of tong associations, the Hong Luck Kung Fu Club's own role was superscribed in several ways. In the earliest days, teaching self-defence to interested members of the Chinatown community had urgency because of the pervasive risk of racially motivated violence.[6] Hong Luck also acted as a de facto security force for some of the tongs by protecting those who could not protect themselves, implementing the associations' justice, and safeguarding their business interests. I witnessed the legacy of this protection role when an elderly, Cantonese-speaking woman came into the club one night asking for Master Paul Chan's assistance in dealing with some local bullies. His reputation in this regard was so established that she did not seem to consider that he was in his late seventies at that point and had long-since relinquished that sort of responsibility. The imperative to train neighbourhood protectors or tong enforcers has diminished over the years, and that aspect of the club now has reduced importance for the Chinatown community at large.

---

[6] Notably, the first non-Chinese Hong Luck member was Métis, followed by an African Canadian. European Canadian members came later, but it appears that the first non-Chinese members were seeking self-defence skills to address racial discrimination like that faced by the club's founders.

As self-defence became less urgent (though still important), some of Hong Luck's fighting spirit went into combat sports such as kickboxing. In the Province of Ontario and surrounding regions, there were several varieties of kickboxing competitions that ranged from light to full contact and from amateur to professional. As sub-category of martial arts, kickboxing is a combat sport that represents the formalization and regulation of older fighting traditions. Thai kickboxing is probably the most well-known variety, with Japanese, Chinese, French, and North American styles also having strong followings. Professional competitors generally wear boxing mitts and minimal protective gear (such as a mouth guard and groin cup), though amateur competitors typically wear more padding. Rules vary in terms of allowable techniques, but all styles involve a combination of punching and kicking between two opponents with a winner determined by points, referee stoppage, or knockout.

Master Paul Chan apparently had some reservations about sport kickboxing because he was more interested in either bare-knuckle self-defence or traditional martial performance. Nonetheless, he still supported students who were more focused on fighting in a ring. Hong Luck has produced several generations of kickboxers. In the early days, competitions typically involved a version of North American kickboxing that included only punches and kicks, with all strikes above the waist. In the 1970s, the McNamara twins discovered Master Paul's rough-and-ready kung fu, which they added to their existing skills in Western boxing and Japanese karate. They later went on to promote kickboxing competitions in Toronto and opened their own franchise of gyms called Twin Dragon Kung Fu and Kickboxing. In the 1980s, Nick Alachiotis had a professional career marked by a high knockout rate; an award plaque still graced the wall of Hong Luck's training hall while I was there. Most recently, Adrian Balcă became a Canadian national Chinese kickboxing gold medallist in 2005.

Chinese kickboxing is typically referred to in English by its Mandarin names, sàndǎ [Cantonese: saandá, 散打], which is literally "scattering strikes," or sànshǒu [Cantonese: saansáu, 散手], which means "scattering hands." Sanda/sanshou was reputedly developed in the early twentieth century by the Chinese military. They conceived of it as hand-to-hand combat training for soldiers, drawing on a mix of the most practical techniques from various styles of kung fu. By the late twentieth century, it had also developed into a combat sport that combines punches and kicks with knee strikes, as well as incorporating wrestling skills like kick-catching, throws, takedowns, and sweeps.

When I started fieldwork at Hong Luck in 2008, practising choreographed "forms" [*toulouh*, 套路] was the most privileged activity,[7] with the requisite stances, attacks, and defences first drilled separately to build a foundation of physical vocabulary for choreography. Most of the weekly classes emphasized preserving the masters' legacies as embodied in forms, which one member estimated at being more than fifty in number. In fact, there was only one class per week dedicated to applications and/or free sparring. To be sure, teachers in the other kung fu classes showed us how the techniques worked, but these explanations were primarily theoretical, and any related exercises relied on a cooperative "opponent." A senior member told me that people needed to know how to use the skills in the forms or else kung fu would run the risk of becoming a dance instead of a martial art. His stance on the meaning of the movement clearly showed the importance of combative function. I observed, however, that Hong Luck members spent most of their time and effort working on the nuances of martial performance, rather than on fighting applications, which is a subtle but important difference. Several senior members assured me that this was the traditional method. Nonetheless, I was sceptical about whether this approach would produce real fighting ability without opportunities to test the skills against a resisting opponent—or at least a partner providing realistic defence. It appeared to me that Hong Luck's training had become superscribed: martial performance was overwriting an older layer of combat application.

Hong Luck members were fiercely proud of their fighting heritage, but there was a tension between their desire to preserve tradition and the evolution of combat training. Since the 1990s, the rising popularity of full-contact mixed martial arts (MMA) competitions like the Ultimate Fighting Championship (UFC) has led hand combat pundits to critique traditional training as being inefficient at best or useless at worst.[8] The argument is that people get good at fighting by practising with a resisting opponent and that they learn how to hit hard by striking focus pads or sand bags. Free sparring

---

[7] Forms were practised in silence at the club but performed in public with martial sound accompaniment from a percussion ensemble, which is a phenomenon I discuss in Chapter 6.

[8] Training against a resisting partner, especially in free-sparring, has long been part of boxing and wrestling in the West, as well as in judo, Thai kickboxing, and taekwondo in the East (among others). The meteoric rise of MMA, however, has shone a spotlight on the effectiveness of martial arts training across styles, because the open format is often billed as "the ultimate proving ground," providing a space for inter-style competition.

(i.e., combat practice without predetermined patterns) can be relatively safe if participants mutually agree on limits to the power of strikes, use protective gear, and apply only "clean" techniques (e.g., no eye pokes or groin strikes). Controlled free sparring allows realistic experience dealing with attack and defence—with reduced risk of serious injury. The traditional training methods I observed at Hong Luck, like non-contact drills and performing choreographed forms, might develop martial skill but not in the most efficient way. In contrast, the combat-sport approach is that to learn to swim, one needs to get in the water.

Apparently, Master Paul had not emphasized sparring because he and the early members got all the fighting experience they needed on the street. During my fieldwork, racial violence was still a concern but no longer a daily one. When kickboxing was more popular, some members recounted having practised free sparring regularly, and they told stories of legendary battles fought in the training hall. During my fieldwork, no one entered any kickboxing tournaments. Without frequent street self-defence against racial violence or the incentive of kickboxing competitions, I observed that Hong Luck members had fewer opportunities to apply their fighting skills. The most practical training I experienced was Hong Luck's weekly sanda kickboxing class, which I attended when my schedule allowed. It varied in intensity depending on who else was there; the free sparring, partner work, and pad training I observed and participated in ranged from mellow to high impact. There were several intermediate and advanced students who attended only that class because they were not interested in forms, lion dance, or percussion, while other members were the opposite. Nonetheless, I observed that people who attended classes in all aspects of the curriculum tended to excel in a holistic way, which is a phenomenon that I address later in the book.

Contested Origins of Traditional Martial Arts in Southern China

The Hong Luck Kung Fu Club has a distinctive tradition based on the individual legacies of Master Paul and Master Jim, but the group's practices are also part of a long collective history of martial arts from China. Far from being straightforward, the origins and development of kung fu lie shrouded by a dense thicket of myths, legends, hagiography, storytelling, literature, drama, ritual, biography, and history. Ultimately, I am most interested in the rich convergence of these factors, although I will tease out some of the strands to consider the plaiting of a metaphorical kung rope.

Not long ago, Stanley Henning called scholarly studies of Chinese martial arts "conspicuous by their relative absence" and disparaged most of what was available (1999: 319). He held up the pioneering kung fu historian Tang Hao [*Tòhng Hòuh*, 唐豪] (1897–1959) as an example, although that author's work remains untranslated and relatively obscure. Similarly, Henning (2006) has sung the praises of contemporary scholars like Ma Mingda, Zhou Weiliang, and Cheng Dali, but their Chinese-language work on martial arts is difficult to access outside of China. In English, historian Peter Lorge (2012) has taken steps to fill the lacuna with a comprehensive historical tome called *Chinese Martial Arts: From Antiquity to the 21st Century*. Political scientist Benjamin Judkins writes an academic blog on Chinese martial studies called *Kung Fu Tea* (chinesemartialstudies.com), and he has also co-authored a book with a narrower focus on the social history of Southern Chinese martial arts in the nineteenth and early twentieth centuries (Judkins and Nielson 2015). While there remains much to do in documenting the history of kung fu, there are now valuable resources in both English and Chinese for balancing myth with fact.

Laypeople—both Eastern and Western—tend to imagine Chinese kung fu as an ancient tradition that blends self-defence with philosophy, but the antiquity and completeness of that blending may not be as it seems. In the popular understanding of Asian martial arts more broadly, one can observe a stance on fighting skills that sees them as tools for performance, sport, and self-cultivation, which has proven useful for promoting martial arts as vehicles for personal development, nation building, and international competition. While appearing ancient, this synthesis is more of an invented tradition (Hobsbawm and Ranger 1983). Peter Lorge argues that privileging anything other than practical technique undermines most of Chinese martial history (2012: 239). Instead, he proposes a view that is more consistent with the bulk of historical practice, which is to regard Chinese martial arts as systems of combat skills that practitioners have sometimes performed for entertainment or ritual purposes (Lorge 2012: 3). Lorge's perspective suggests that kung fu is basically about training to fight, representing the evolution and codification of techniques used by both soldiers and civilians in battle. Viewed this way, ritual, spiritual, theatrical, or sporting expressions of martial skills might have important pedigrees of their own in China, but they do not form the core of "real" kung fu. A combative orientation also affects the way people hear martial sound. From this standpoint, the gong and drum ensemble used in kung fu and lion dance maintains the legacy of the instruments used to signal troop movements in ancient warfare.

By recognizing the important role of folk history in the martial arts, other scholars are more interested in how stories construct meaning and perhaps even change the past. Anthropologist Thomas A. Green (2003), for example, does not concern himself with the accuracy of kung fu tales, but rather looks at how practitioners use them to establish credibility, present parables, encourage a mind-set of resistance, and/or build group pride. In this sense, combat systems were superscribed with imaginative narratives in order to elevate them to the level of being martial arts of self-cultivation. In so doing, kung fu came to draw heavily on stories about mythical founders, superscribing the fighting skills with layers of meaning related to spirituality and even imbuing the techniques with mystical energies.

There is also a case to be made for kung fu as we know it having more to do with performance and ritual than fighting, which is a rather more modern perspective than that of Peter Lorge. As historian Charles Holcombe writes:

> In China the martial arts are an aspect of religion, with all of the attendant mystery and miracles. At the same time, the public face of the martial arts has often been that of the entertainer, and the self-image of the martial artist has been thoroughly imbued with motifs drawn from fiction and the theatre. (2002: 166)

Contemporary kung fu owes much to the heterodox religious sects and secret societies that arose in eighteenth- and nineteenth-century China, as I will discuss in the next section. Popularity among the illiterate and semi-literate masses relied on cloaking ideology in the characters, stories, and heroic atmosphere of popular theatre, storytelling, and folk religion. Holcombe (2002) argues that today's Chinese martial arts owe more to this religious and dramatic base than to a tradition of real fighting skills. From this perspective, gong and drum ensembles in kung fu and lion dance are an extension of religious, ritual, and operatic percussion in China.

I will not try to resolve the debate on the origins of "authentic" Chinese martial arts because any such effort is doomed to fail. The complexities of the subject matter simply do not allow a totalizing definition. China is a huge country with a recorded martial history of over 3,000 years. There are reputedly over a hundred distinct styles of Chinese martial arts being practised in the twenty-first century, both within Greater China and in the diaspora. Even practitioners of the same type of kung fu often have very different approaches based on their own lineages, personalities, and abilities. As a result, I will provide a history for Hong Luck's kung fu that respects its complex, diverse, and contested origins, while also giving a useable context to the specific practices I have encountered during my fieldwork.

The Choi Lee Fut and Do Pi Styles of Kung Fu

During my fieldwork, the Hong Luck Kung Fu Club's curriculum focused on two styles of Chinese martial arts: Choi Lee Fut and Do Pi. They both have their origins in Southern China's Guangdong Province, although they arose at different times and locations. While these were the two main styles, they were not the only ones. Over the course of half a century in Toronto, the club's tradition became a syncretic blend of not only the martial arts that the founders learned as youths in Taishan, but also ones they picked up in Hong Kong before coming to Canada, as well as others that they learned on later trips back to China or from visiting masters who taught at Hong Luck over the years. Furthermore, Choi Lee Fut and Do Pi are themselves syncretic, and practitioners openly acknowledge the blending of sources from older styles. Even within Choi Lee Fut, there are different branches, several of which I encountered during my fieldwork at Hong Luck. As a result, the tradition that I met included a cross-section of many of the major Southern Chinese kung fu styles. A Chinese model of tradition as "source and stream" [*yùhn làuh*, 源流] is a helpful metaphor here, which Stephen Jones (1996) has drawn on to describe the relationship between early music and living tradition in China. The regional similarities of Southern Chinese martial arts systems allowed them to circulate together within the club, acting as tributaries of Hong Luck's river. On the one hand, diverse tributaries flow into the river of tradition and merge together. On the other, a watercourse cut off from its source will eventually dry up and die.

Choi Lee Fut is the older of Hong Luck's two main styles. Its origins go back to the Xinhui [*Sānwúi*, 新會] district of Guangdong in the 1830s. The founder of the system was Chan Heung [*Chàhn Hēung Jóusī*, 陳享祖師] (circa 1806–1875). He named Choi Lee Fut in honour of the three styles that he combined: Choi Family boxing a.k.a. Choi Gar [*Choi Gā kyùhn*, 蔡家

拳], Lee Family boxing a.k.a. Lee Gar [*Léih Gā kyùhn*, 李家拳], and Buddha boxing a.k.a. Fut Gar [*Faht Gā kyùhn*, 佛家拳] (Lee 1983).[9] Chan's new style spread throughout Guangdong as his disciples opened branch schools; it became the most widely practised martial art in the province until its decline after the end of the Chinese Civil War in 1949 (Judkins and Nielson 2015: 92). As one of the first franchised martial arts in China's emerging modern era, Choi Lee Fut's success was in part a response to the grave political uncertainties created by wars and rebellions. The Qing Dynasty was decaying and local militias were becoming a necessity in Guangdong, so training in hand combat for civilians was a high priority (Judkins and Nielson 2015: 94). Thanks to its syncretic origins, Choi Lee Fut has a rich array of armed and unarmed fighting techniques for dealing with diverse combative situations, which helped fuel its popularity in China during the nineteenth and early twentieth centuries. Thereafter, the style spread around the world with Cantonese migrants.

Over time, Choi Lee Fut has fragmented into several different lineages. In their youths, both Masters Paul and Jim learned village styles of Choi Lee Fut in Taishan.[10] Towards the end of his life, however, Master Paul was promoting a mainstream interpretation of Choi Lee Fut, which he had been learning on return trips to China. This version of the style enjoyed emerging support from local authorities in the PRC. Such support is significant because the Chinese Communist Party suppressed traditional kung fu for many years, particularly during the Cultural Revolution (1966–1976). Master Paul's stance on standardization recognized the value of aligning Hong Luck's brand with Guangdong's provincial sporting mandate in order to connect the club to larger organizations. Despite Master Paul's efforts to emphasize mainstream Choi Lee Fut towards the end of his life, it is only one part of Hong Luck's history and tradition. In fact, even the standardized Choi Lee Fut forms that he brought back from China became not so standard once Hong Luck members started practising them.

---

[9] The Chinese character used in the name of many styles of kung fu literally means "fist" and metaphorically means "boxing" [Cantonese: *kyùhn*, 拳], but it is a metonym for martial arts styles that also include other techniques, e.g., kicking, grappling, and/or weapons. The same character appears in the naming of choreographed forms, e.g., Small Plum Flower Boxing [*Síu Múihfā Kyùhn*, 小梅花拳].

[10] The Taishan Choi Lee Fut taught at Hong Luck is a "short-bridge" [*dyún kìuh*, 短橋] style, meaning it focuses on close- and medium-range striking, although it also has long-range attacks. In contrast, mainstream Choi Lee Fut is "long-bridge" [*chèuhng kìuh*, 長橋], meaning it focuses on the longer ranges of combat. In Chinese kung fu, the arms are called "bridges" [*kìuh sáu*, 橋手] because they join opponents together during a fight.

In contrast to the prominence of Choi Lee Fut, Do Pi is less well known. The founder Chan Dau [*Chàhn Dau Jóusī*, 陳斗祖師] established his first training hall in the city of Guangzhou during the 1920s, later moving to Hong Kong in 1932 (Lee n.d.). This timeline makes Do Pi approximately a hundred years younger than Choi Lee Fut. Both styles are hybrids of other types of Southern kung fu. Do Pi includes Choi Lee Fut within it as well as Hung Family boxing a.k.a. Hung Gar [*Hùhng Gā kyùhn*, 洪家拳], Chow Family boxing a.k.a. Jow Gar [*Jāu Gā kyùhn*, 周家拳],[11] and Knight Style boxing a.k.a. Hop Gar [*Hahp Gā kyùhn* 俠家拳]. Chan Dau was also open to non-Chinese styles, incorporating influences from the Western boxing that his Hung Gar teacher had learned in the United States before returning to China (Lee n.d.). The martial character of Do Pi differs from Choi Lee Fut in that it is more streamlined and aggressive. Master Paul studied with Chan Dau in Hong Kong. Back in Toronto, his stance on Do Pi emphasized its practicality. Master Paul was known for his forward pressure when he fought, epitomizing a Do Pi method called "colliding and beating" [*johng dá*, 撞打].

Apart from the two main styles, there are three other currents still circulating strongly through Hong Luck.[12] First, as I mentioned previously, kickboxing has long had a following at the club. In an era when self-defence on the street has become intermittent, sparring has helped maintain fighting traditions and vivify choreographed forms by giving practitioners experience with applied technique. Second, instructors taught a village style of Hung Gar in the club's early days, which continues to inform Hong Luck's basic training with an emphasis on deep, wide, stable stances that exceeds what is normally seen in either Choi Lee Fut or Do Pi. Case in point, my lion dance teachers asserted that Hung Gar footwork was essential to Hong Luck's style of dancing. Third, Master Jim studied Northern Style [*Bāk Paai*, 北派] alongside Choi Lee Fut when he was a boy. Like Southern Chinese kung fu, there are many distinct styles of martial arts from Northern China, but Master Jim only ever referred to what he had learned in a general way. The Northern Style forms he taught had a more extended, florid, and theatrical quality than his practical, economical, and combative Choi Lee Fut, contributing to some of Hong Luck's most crowd-pleasing choreography and informing all the club's

[11] Jow Gar is also a hybrid, sometimes described as "Hung head with Choi tail" [*Hùhng tàuh Choi méih*, 洪頭蔡尾] because it fuses Hung Gar and Choi Gar.

[12] Many members trained in other martial arts too numerous to list, whether before or during their time at Hong Luck. Examples of the other repertoire included Japanese karate, Western boxing, and Russian sambo, as well as Chinese styles like Fut Gar and tai chi [*taai gihk kyùhn*, 太極拳].

performances. Additionally, Master Paul had studied Japanese judo, and it was once a formal part of the club's curriculum. By the time I arrived at Hong Luck, judo was no longer practised with any regularity, although vestiges of it remained in the odd technique like a break-fall or throw. These varied influences from other styles could not help but affect Hong Luck's Choi Lee Fut and Do Pi, providing grounds for comparison and contrast.

With so many different styles and influences circulating at Hong Luck, I found it remarkable that members took such a firmly traditional stance on their martial arts. Despite the obvious syncretism, it was meaningful to them that they endeavoured to preserve and pass on what their teachers taught them—and thus what their teachers' teachers had taught, and so on. Nonetheless, each generation of practitioners has added their own experiences, superscribing the received tradition with new meanings while never quite erasing the old ones. For example, Master Paul's beloved Do Pi was created in the 1930s when Chan Dau fused the Jow, Choi Lee Fut, Hung, and Hop styles. These styles became united like tributaries merging into a larger watercourse, and yet there remains a Confucian respect for the older sources as ancestors. In fact, the aforementioned source and stream process (Jones 1996) is referenced in the couplet of Chinese characters on the wall at Hong Luck that frame the Do Pi founder's photo (see Figure 2.1). The short poem emphasizes a "true transmission" from the "streaming sources." I have translated the couplet below, with added bold to show the characters I am referring to.

> The family of the Way's **true transmission** of fist, staff, and cudgel
> [*douh gā **jān chyùhn** kyùhn gwan páahng*, 道家真傳拳棍棒];
> The faction's **streaming sources** of sword, knife, and spear
> [*paai haih **làuh yùhn** gīm dōu chēung*, 派系流源劍刀槍].

For context, it is also worth noting that the city of Toronto has a long history of martial arts and combat sports, so Hong Luck's members have always-already operated in a melting pot of physical culture. In the early twenty-first century, nearly every style of hand combat imaginable can be practised in multicultural Toronto, but I will outline some trends in popularity over time. Western pugilism and fencing were brought over by British settlers and were well established by the end of the nineteenth century. Japanese karate and judo were the first Asian martial arts to spread outside their ethnic community, and they became widely practised beginning in the middle of the

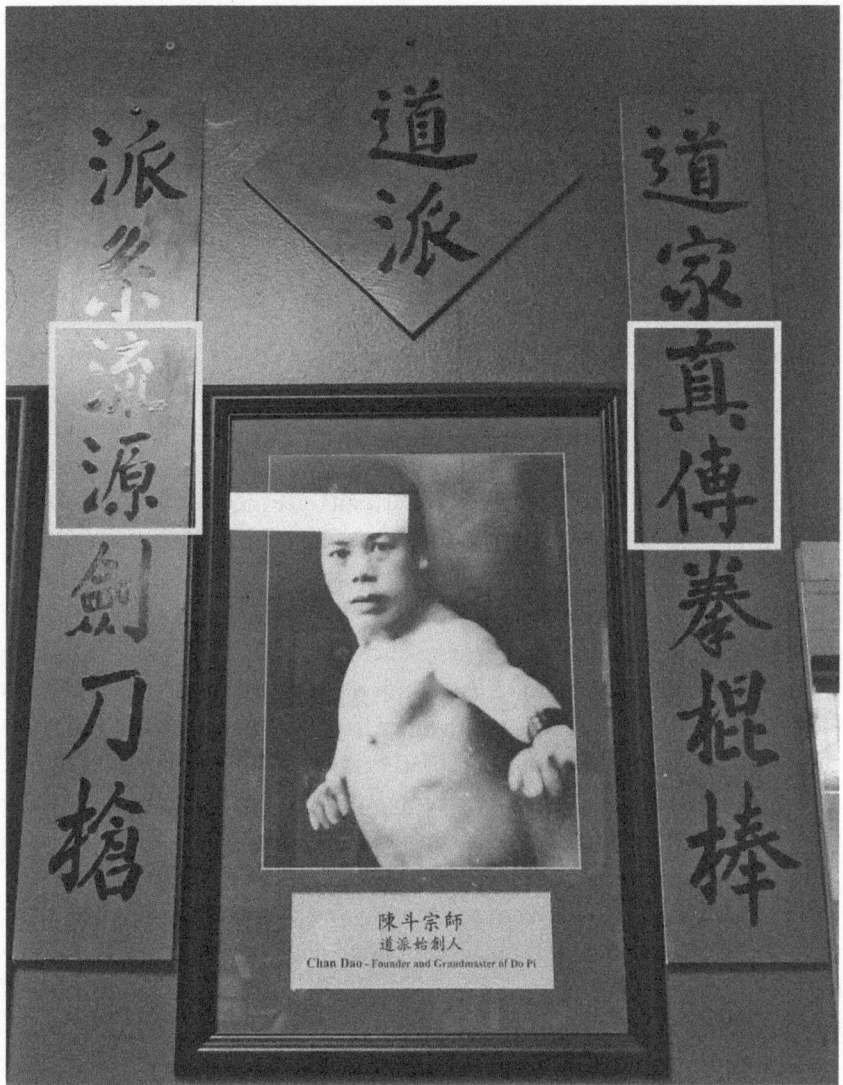

Figure 2.1 Do Pi couplet [*Douh Paai deuilyùhn*, 道派對聯]
Credits: Colin P. McGuire

twentieth century. According to my fieldwork consultants, Chinese kung fu remained more of a closed community until the meteoric rise to fame of actor Bruce Lee in the 1970s, at which point Hong Luck's classes were filled to bursting with eager students. The current popularity of MMA was launched by the UFC in the early 1990s, with its novel idea of a fighting competition open to all styles. MMA continues to enjoy the lion's share of mainstream popularity, and gyms specializing in admixtures of Brazilian jujitsu, Thai kickboxing, as well as Western boxing and wrestling have proliferated like mushrooms after a rainstorm. In a way, Master Paul was ahead of his time when he began incorporating judo's grappling skills with kung fu striking, although he never competed in a ring or cage. At the same time, his approach builds on the legacies of Choi Lee Fut and Do Pi, both of which are themselves blends of other styles.

The Story/History of the Shaolin Temple

Although Hong Luck's profusion of kung fu lineages may seem complicated, there is a common thread: these martial arts all trace their roots to the famous Shaolin Temple [*Siulàhm Jí*, 少林寺]. In fact, most styles of Cantonese martial arts do the same. No history of martial arts in Southern China is therefore complete without a discussion of Shaolin,[13] which is a Gordian knot of stories and histories. Practitioners and aficionados typically claim that kung fu was born in the Shaolin Buddhist temple on Mount Song in central China's Henan Province during the late fifth and early sixth centuries. Ironically, the credit for inventing Chinese martial arts goes to Bodhidharma, an Indian monk who is also believed to have brought Buddhism to China, becoming the first patriarch of the Chan sect [Cantonese: *Sihm*, 禪, Japanese: Zen]. As the essential version of the story goes, he felt his disciples at Shaolin were too weak to endure long periods of meditation and were also vulnerable to attack. Bodhidharma taught them a set of boxing movements for self-defence and meditative calisthenics for health, which became the foundation of Chinese kung fu.

Evidence-based scholars have disparaged this tale of kung fu's Shaolin origins as a gross distortion, if not outright fabrication (Henning 1999; Lorge 2012). Historical sources show that boxing, wrestling, weapons, martial dances, and Chinese Buddhism all predate the Shaolin Temple. The idea of mixing martial arts with introspection, however, is more recent. A connection between fighting skills and Taoist self-cultivation exercises first arose towards the end of the Ming Dynasty (1368–1644 CE), which coincides

---

[13] In Southern China, not all martial arts are Cantonese, and Hakka people in Guangdong (a distinct ethnic sub-group) do not typically subscribe to Shaolin mythology (see Judkins and Nielson 2015).

with the first recorded claim that Bodhidharma was the originator of kung fu (Shahar 2008: 165–172). The Bodhidharma-as-founder kung fu myth appears to have become fully entrenched only in the early twentieth century, thanks to serialized martial arts novels (Henning 1999).

As with the best tales, there is a grain of truth to the stories about Shaolin. During the Ming Dynasty, martial culture was in decline among both elite rulers and the hereditary warrior class, but Shaolin had its own private army (Shahar 2008: 4). Significantly, this army occasionally provided military assistance to the Ming emperor, thus earning the temple a patriotic reputation. Shaolin warrior monks and lay disciples were most well known for pole-fighting skills. In the tolerant and relatively open atmosphere of the late Ming, however, Shaolin monks also began developing martial arts with less directly military applications. They did so as participants in the broader trends of the era, synthesizing related, but previously separate, traditions of martial arts and meditation. Another Ming trend was reworking generic types of boxing, grappling, and weapons into distinctive styles of hand combat. Combined with the interdisciplinary idea of infusing martial arts with meditation, these new systems had a novel approach that simultaneously trained fighting, performance, and self-cultivation.

The primacy of Shaolin as the source of martial arts has more to do with hagiography than it does originality. The monks from Mount Song may not have done it first, but they did it best (or at least most famously), which changed the story to attribute innovation to them. It is common practice in Chinese literature and philosophy to attach new ideas to ancient origins in order to lend them validity within a Confucian value structure whose stance on legitimacy privileges the old. The creation of historical narratives can thus occur in a non-chronological way. For example, the figure of Guan Yu became linked to Buddhism when the faith was under attack from the Confucian establishment (Duara 1988: 778–779). A story recorded in 820 CE about an event from centuries before claimed that Guan Yu's restless ghost found peace through learning about karma, thereby establishing him as a Buddhist tutelary deity.[14] Guan Yu already held the respect of Confucians, so this story served to retroactively superscribe Buddhism with his virtues.

A widely known story explains how civilians began practising Shaolin martial arts. After Manchurians invaded China from the north and established

---

[14] In Buddhism, the word *karma* means the influence of good and bad deeds on one's situation, in this life as well as after reincarnation.

the Qing Dynasty in 1644, they feared Shaolin's martial heritage and loyalty to the defeated Ming Dynasty. Not long after, the Qing army burned down a Shaolin Temple for fear that Shaolin might become involved in rebellion. Three martial monks, one warrior nun, and a lay disciple escaped from the fire; they collectively became known as the Five Elders [Ńgh Jóu, 五祖]. The escapees fled south to Guangdong Province and began teaching their fighting skills to laypeople, thereby founding many of the major styles of Southern kung fu. For example, the three styles that Chan Heung combined to form Choi Lee Fut all trace their lineages back to one of the Five Elders, a Buddhist master named Jee Shin [Jisìhn Sìhmsī, 至善禪師]. There are many versions of this tale. In some, another layer of myth superscribes the legend with a Shaolin Temple in Southern China's Fujian Province, instead of the original one in Henan Province. Despite the claims of folk history, there is a lack of empirical evidence for the existence of a branch in Fujian (Shahar 2008: 184). Nonetheless, the core of the Five Shaolin Elders story remains consistent, even if the details may shift from version to version.

Shaolin kung fu origin stories helped legitimize the accelerating proliferation of Chinese martial arts styles in the eighteenth and nineteenth centuries. Many martial artists at the time were itinerant, living at the margins of society and working as caravan security, mercenary militiamen, bodyguards for hire, Cantonese opera artists, wandering teachers, or street-market martial arts performers (Kennedy and Guo 2005: 144–146). They lived in an underworld known as "rivers and lakes" [gōngwùh, 江湖] (Boretz 2011: 31–37).[15] For many of the new kung fu styles, it was good for business to superscribe older meanings through a connection to the famous Shaolin Temple; it helped attract clients, students, and audiences.

Ming-loyalist secret societies also used stories about Five Elders, albeit with their own slightly different set of variations (Murray and Qin 1994). The most important of these groups for kung fu purposes was the Heaven and Earth Society [Tīndeihwuí, 天地會].[16] Historical records show that they began as a multi-surname mutual aid association in Fujian Province in the early 1760s, not as Ming-loyalist rebels (Murray and Qin 1994). At the time, mutual aid groups were prevalent, responding to the economic and political instabilities of the era. The Heaven and Earth Society eventually spread with migrants throughout Southern China and the diaspora, expanding to

---

[15] The Mandarin term for the world of rivers and lakes is jiānghú, which has gained some currency in English thanks to its use in films but is not (yet) found in standard dictionaries.

[16] The Mandarin for Heaven and Earth Society is Tiāndì Huì.

participate in widely different activities, including not only mutual aid and protection, but also predatory crime and sedition.[17] It was not until later that the Heaven and Earth Society developed a Ming-loyalist origin myth attached to the burning of the Shaolin Temple (ter Haar 2000). Given some of the Heaven and Earth Society's more questionable activities, a Shaolin affiliation would certainly have been good for public relations, but the religious overtones also helped with group cohesion. According to David Ownby (1995), the merging of mutual-aid structures with popular religion was a key factor in the success of Southern Chinese secret societies; the origin myth helped deepen a stance on loyalty when members swore blood oaths upon joining.

Again, I wish to emphasize that martial arts schools were related to, but separate from, religion, mutual aid, and rebellion. Judkins and Nielsen suggest that the organizational structure of kung fu clubs most closely resembles that of merchant guilds, which centred on skills development (2015: 101). Nineteenth-century anti-Qing secret societies and Shaolin-descended kung fu groups appear to have influenced each other and sometimes even had an overlapping membership, hence why both types of groups used Shaolin to superscribe their activities with historical and cultural value. The legacy of mutual influences between Cantonese kung fu styles and the Heaven and Earth Society persists in the way that Choi Lee Fut practitioners talk about their lineages. Two of the largest branches of the style are both called Hung Sing, although they use different Chinese characters for the word *hung*. As the stories go, Choi Lee Fut was an anti-Qing martial art—or at least some practitioners sympathized with a rebel ideology. Another name for the Heaven and Earth Society was the *Hùhngmùhn* [洪門], which is literally a "big/deluge gate," but it translates as the Hung League, where Hung is a family name. Kung fu styles wishing to disguise their allegiance to "victory of the Hung" [*Hùhng Sing,* 洪勝], while still referencing it for other insiders, would come to use a homophonous character when naming their styles. Hong Luck is a Hung Sing [*Hùhng Sing,* 雄勝] Choi Lee Fut club, while the New Asia Kung Fu Society that I trained with in Hong Kong uses the other way of writing it [*Hùhng Sing,* 鴻勝]. The former means something like "mighty/grand victory," while the latter is "vast/huge victory."

---

[17] In some cases, the Heaven and Earth Society has been associated with organized crime a.k.a. the Triads.

Despite the absence of evidence for kung fu as we know it having literally come from the Five Elders, the Shaolin legend remains a powerfully mean- ingful phenomenon. The Manchurians who established the Qing Dynasty were foreign invaders from beyond China's borders, so Shaolin's histor- ical military support of the Ming Dynasty empowered mythmaking that resulted in a stance on the intrinsic Chinese-ness of kung fu. Qing Dynasty Manchurians were a distinct ethnic group, separate from the Han people who had controlled the Ming Dynasty. The vast majority of Chinese people then (as now) were Han and considered themselves to be the original inhabitants of China. The (in)famous rebel motto was "overthrow the Qing, restore the Ming" [fáan Chīng fuhk Mìhng, 反清復明], which implies returning China to Han control. Chinese people thus held Shaolin as not only a source of fighting skills, but also a symbol of allegiance to the Chinese-ness of the Ming. Through Shaolin, kung fu came to embody an ethos of resistance to oppression, while offering a distinctly Chinese way of being-in-the-world.

Practically speaking, guns had already superseded hand combat in China since the mid-1800s (Worthing 2007: 60), so serious revolutionaries would have been unlikely to dally with the more esoteric hand-to-hand fighting methods of kung fu. Nonetheless, the spirit of resistance embodied in Shaolin connections may have kept the flame of revolution alive. Shaolin ide- ology influenced the way kung fu practitioners thought of their martial arts, shaping them regardless of whether the practices originated in that temple. A stance of resistance to the Qing made secret societies more appealing as they competed to build their strength through numbers. In most cases, how- ever, Shaolin resistance was more symbolic than literal until actual revolu- tionary leaders like Sun Yat-sen harnessed secret societies to support real rebellion (DeKorne 1934).

After the Qing Dynasty fell in 1911, the nascent Republic of China led by the Kuomintang deployed empowering rhetoric focused on modernization and rebuilding. You see, it was not just the work of revolutionaries that led to the end of imperial rule, because the incursion of foreign powers and the Qing's internal decay played significant roles as well. The new leaders sought to rid themselves of the damning title, "sick man of East Asia" [Dūng Aa bèhng fū, 東亞病夫]. Nationalist leaders and martial arts reformers alike fo- cused on becoming able to compete in Western sports, as well as mass partic- ipation in calisthenics, as means of national "self-strengthening" [jih kèuhng, 自強]. After nearly a century of ongoing domination by European powers and Imperialist Japan, the fledgling Republic of China sought to build up the bodies of its people as the root of a strong, modern nation. The stance on physical strength was that it would empower the body politic to resist imperialist incursions.

Some reformers still recognized the value of kung fu and promoted a new approach to martial arts training. As documented by Andrew Morris (2004) in his history of Republican China's rapidly evolving physical culture, both private groups and governmental agencies went to work rehabilitating the marginalized image of kung fu. During this time, Chinese martial arts became known as "national arts" [*gwokseuht*, 國術] as a way of strengthening the populace through activities with embedded cultural roots (Kennedy and Guo 2005: 102–113). Modernization efforts aimed to do away with outdated training methods and to eliminate superstitious beliefs, while still preserving kung fu heritage. The failed Boxer Uprising [*Yihwòh Tyùhn Wahnduhng*, 義和團運動] of 1898 is a prime example of the excesses that reformers were targeting. In Northern China, the Boxers had promoted a blend of heterodox religion with martial arts that led adherents to believe they were invulnerable to bullets, which obviously no amount of kung fu training can make possible.[18]

After the Chinese Civil War ended (1927–1950), the victorious Chinese Communist Party (CCP) also recognized the value of martial arts but promoted a more radical approach to reform. By 1965, the People's Physical Culture and Sports Commission had created national rules and compulsory routines for competition (Henning 1981), resulting in state-sponsored, standardized, Chinese martial arts as sporting performance. Traditional kung fu was once again pushed to the margins of society and was even the target of violent purges during the Cultural Revolution (1967–1976). The military continued to practise the sanda kickboxing that I mentioned earlier, but the new CCP vision for Chinese martial arts emphasized splitting the blurred genre of kung fu into separate categories of martial performance and combat sport, so performers did not fight and fighters did not perform. It was not until after the Cultural Revolution that interdisciplinary kung fu began to make a comeback in China, although by that point many traditional masters had already been forced to stop practising, passed away, or emigrated. Hong Luck's co-founding masters thus have a fairly common story of leaving

---

[18] Ironically, the Boxers supported the Qing, but their attacks on foreigners and Chinese Christians hastened the dynasty's end. Collateral damage from the fighting and reparations owed to the Western nations who crushed the uprising further weakened an already floundering Qing.

China and preserving their kung fu in diaspora during a time when they might not have been able to do so in their homeland.

Most traditional Southern Chinese kung fu styles, like those practised at Hong Luck, continue to connect with Shaolin as a matter of identity, not religion or verifiable lineage. It is more the idea of Shaolin that pervades the club, fostering an ethos of Chinese-ness and resistance to oppression. At Hong Luck, members mentioned Shaolin as the source of Chinese kung fu, but they did not teach the origin story as part of the club's curriculum. Instead, members' knowledge on the subject appeared to have come from popular media like movies, TV, magazines, books, and the internet. For example, internationally famous kung fu movies like 1982's *The Shaolin Temple*, starring Jet Li [*Léih Lìhn-giht*, 李連傑], have uncritically reinforced the legends. There is plenty of Buddhist symbolism built into Hong Luck's martial arts, especially in the names of forms and techniques, but the stance on day-to-day practice was largely secular. When Hong Luck members were involved in rituals like lion dancing or lighting incense at Guan Yu's altar, these practices were not expressions of formal religious Buddhism, but rather a form of the Chinese popular folk-religion sometimes called the Three Teachings [*Sāam Gaau*, 三教], which blends Confucianism, Taoism, and Buddhism (Harrell 1977; Yang and Hu 2012).

Origins and Symbolism of Lion Dance

Lions are not native to China, and yet the lion dance has become an important symbol for Chinese people, especially in the diaspora. Although there are historical records of a Chinese emperor receiving a living lion as a gift from a neighbouring country some 2,000 years ago, the more important and widespread influence on lion dancing is probably the use of these big cats in Buddhist iconography (Liu 1981: 15). Asiatic lions are native to India (the birthplace of the historical Buddha, Siddhārtha Gautama), where religious art depicts them as ferocious guardians of Buddhist truth. As Buddhism spread throughout China, this image spread with it and took on a life beyond its original use. Pairs of "lion statues" [*sehk sī*, 石獅] became common outside doorways as guardians of not only temples, but also tombs, palaces, and eventually homes and businesses.[19] As with the Cantonese lion dance

---

[19] In English, guardian lion statues are sometimes erroneously called *foo dogs*.

costumes, these "lion" statues are often exaggerated or even fantastical in their appearance, rather than being an accurate representation of natural cats (see Figure 2.2).

The earliest descriptions of lion dance are from the Tang Dynasty (618–907 CE), but the practice likely evolved from the ancient tradition of mimetic animal dances going back to the Zhou Dynasty (1045–256 BCE) (Liu 1981: 31). The Tang lion was a court dance that embodied the Chinese philosophies of "five elements" [*ńgh hàhng*, 五行], "five directions" [*ńgh fōng*, 五方], and "five virtues" [*ńgh sèuhng*, 五常] through colour, number of lions, and spatial positioning (Hu 1995: 67–68).[20] It also incorporated Buddhist symbolism and dramatic commentary on political events of the time (Liu 1981: 33). The lion costume featured a carved wooden head attached to a cloth body animated by two people. In the *Official History of the Tang Dynasty* (舊唐書, cited in Hu 1995: 69), there is a description of a 140-man chorus accompanying five dancing lions by singing a tune called "Peace and Security Music" [*Taaipìhng Ngohk*, 太平樂]. Hu adds that there were also musicians playing wind, string, and percussion instruments. Unfortunately, we have no music notation to describe these performances, which is likely because imperial scholars tended not to bother documenting entertainment genres (Thrasher 2008: 53). When detachments of the military went on campaign, they brought the lion dance with them and performed it in public, albeit in a less grandiose way than at the height of the Tang court (Hu 1995: 4, 107). In this way, a dance that originated as a refined, philosophical entertainment for the nobility reached the common people.

The Tang Dynasty was a golden age for Chinese civilization, and so attributing the contemporary lion dance's origins to that time is compelling for practitioners because of the respect it entails. For example, William C. C. Hu was a scholar, a lion dancer, and member of Honolulu, Hawai'i's Chinese Physical Culture Association [*Wàh Yàhn Jīng Móuh Táiyuhk Wúi*, 華人精武體育會] (1995: 334), which may have influenced the way his seminal English-language book on lion dance sometimes reads like a lineage story.[21] Making connections going back to the Tang Dynasty occurs in other places as well,

[20] The five elements are: water, earth, wood, metal, and fire. The five directions are: east, south, west, north, and centre. The five virtues are: benevolence, righteousness, propriety, wisdom, and fidelity.
[21] Hu's book, *Chinese Lion Dance Explained* (1995), is long out of print, but it may still be found in some libraries. When copies are available for purchase, I have seen them command exorbitant prices. It is an important resource because it contains an immense amount of cultural and historical information, albeit with a lack critical perspective on the author's own subject position.

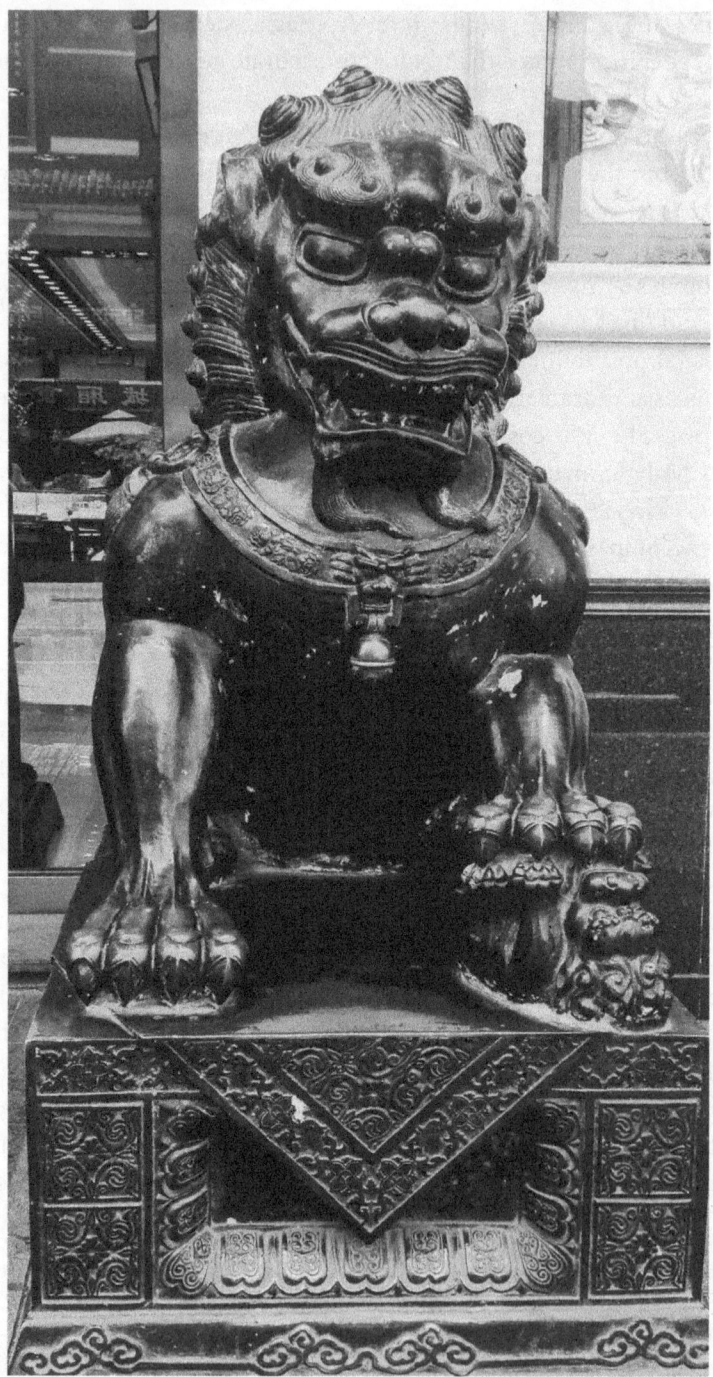

Figure 2.2 Guardian lion statue
Credits: Colin P. McGuire

such as Toronto's Chinatown (and many others in diaspora) being known as Tang People Street [*Tòhng Yàhn Gāai*, 唐人街]. Echoing Bodhidharma's founding of kung fu at Shaolin during the Tang Dynasty, the claiming of heritage from that era is also found in other genres of expressive culture from China. The chamber musics of both the Chaozhou and Minnan peoples of Southern China claim direct Tang provenance (Thrasher 2008: 7–14). Alan Thrasher cautions, however, that questions of origin are problematic, having been complicated by more than a millennium of intervening history (2008: 14). Interestingly, in both lion dance and the "southern pipes" music [Mandarin: *nánguǎn*, Cantonese: *nàahmgún*, 南管] of Fujian and Taiwan, clannish groups with primarily amateur, rural/working-class membership trace their practices back to the glorious Tang Dynasty (Chou 2002). Such a move shows a stance on respect for ancient things, hanging contemporary practice on an ancient pedigree to enhance its prestige. When I spoke with my teachers about the origins of lion dance, they told me that it was very old, but they did not know when it started. There is a Tang Dynasty origin story on Hong Luck's website, however, which credits an unnamed emperor with inventing the lion dance.

During the Song Dynasty (960–1126 CE), a martial arts master in Zhejiang Province named Yang Hsien-ch'iang [*Yèuhng Hín-chēung*, 楊顯槍] is credited with adapting the courtly lion dance of the Tang Dynasty to further enhance its entertainment value for the masses (Hu 1995: 116–117). He did away with the heavy wooden mask of the Tang, substituting a lighter one made from papier-mâché over a bamboo frame. This innovation allowed dancers to infuse the sedate court dance with martial vigour, displaying leaps, kicks, and balances. His other innovation was musical in nature:

> Earlier, various musical instrumentations of percussion, wind, string and song were utilized. However, Master Yang Hsien-ch'iang was only familiar with military drumming so he used only percussion instruments of drums, gongs and cymbals. Moreover, the rhythmic patterns of drumming imitated the military style for the various signalling of troops. (Hu 1995: 120)

William Hu refers to Yang Hsien-ch'iang as a *martial artist* (1995: 116), but this is hundreds of years before the emergence of kung fu styles as we know them today (as described earlier in this chapter). Given the reference to military drumming in the quote above, Yang may have been a former soldier. His contributions would be an important evolutionary step between the

Tang court lion dance and that of contemporary kung fu groups, but I hesitate to take the story literally. The Baidu Baike Chinese wiki-style encyclopedia entry on the "yellow sand lion" [*wòhng sā sījí*, 黃沙獅子] of the Song Dynasty refers to Yang Hsien-ch'iang as "legend/folklore" [*chyùhnsyut*, 傳說].[22] As with Shaolin, we might understand this story as a valid folk explanation of the lion dance's martial stance, which does not necessarily have (or need) historical veracity.

By the Ming Dynasty, common people in Anhui Province were using the lion dance during New Year's ceremonies (Liu 1981: 35). The fearsome look of the mask and its superscribed role as a protector in Buddhist iconography merged to give the meaning of an exorcism ritual. In performance, the combination of a frightening mask, vigorous movement, and thunderous percussion dispelled negative energies, which paved the way for health, happiness, and prosperity to flourish. As the New Year period is a point of renewal and the start of another cycle, such preparations were—and are—important to people's life-worlds. The same ritual logic continues to apply in contemporary lion dancing, as exemplified by the Hong Luck Kung Fu Club's annual New Year parade through their local Chinatown.

Hong Luck's old website contained several legends regarding the origins of the lion dance. Nonetheless, I never heard members telling these tales around the club, nor did anyone suggest any legendary explanations when I asked about the origins of lion dance. That is to say, these origin myths were not part of Hong Luck's oral tradition. Instead, they came from broader lion dance culture; the group of senior members who created the website collected the stories from books, magazines, and the internet in order to generate added-value content. The myths on the site are like those collected by other lion dance researchers (Hu 1995; Liu 1981; Slovenz-Low 1994), and I will quote Hong Luck's version at length here:

> A popular belief is that the lion dance finds its roots in the Tang Dynasty (AD 618–906). Legend has it that the emperor had a strange dream one night. In his dream, an odd creature he had never laid eyes upon before saved his life and carried him to safety. The next day, wondering what this creature was and what the dream meant, the emperor described his reverie to his ministers. One of the ministers explained that the strange creature resembled an animal called a "lion," which did not exist in China at the

---

[22] https://baike.baidu.com/item/黃沙獅子 (accessed 21 February 2018).

time. The emperor, wanting to see this "lion" while awake, ordered them to create a model of it, and because of his dream, the lion came to symbolize good luck, happiness, and prosperity.

Another account tells of a lion frequently terrorising a small village in China. In order to stop the attacks of the beast, all the villagers banded together and beat their pots and pans to make a racket that could drive away the lion. It is said some even put on costumes that resembled the lion. Other versions of this account tell of the villagers consulting a Buddhist monk for protection. The monk eventually tamed the lion, which in turn became the protector of the people. This monk is often represented as a big - headed Buddha (dai to fut), as seen in most Southern lion dances.

Probably, the most credible version of the origin of the lion dance is this. of a [sic] mythical lion originating in heaven was reborn. Being very mischievous and having a fondness for practical jokes, he created a great deal of trouble for everyone. On one occasion, he decided to play a practical joke on the Jade Emperor. Angered at the trouble the lion caused, the Jade Emperor killed the lion by cutting the lion's head off and separating it from its body. He then threw both the head and the body of the lion down to the earth to rot. Upon discovering the fate of the lion, Kwan Yin (the goddess of mercy) felt sorry for the lion and decided to help him. Using a long red ribbon, she tied the lions head back on and brought him back to life. This red ribbon is still seen today, and is said to have the ability to ward off the evil spirits. Kwan Yin also adorned the lion with a horn and mirror to drive away evil spirits.[23]

Hong Luck's lion dance has its strongest historical roots in the late Qing Dynasty. Nineteenth-century martial arts groups in Guangdong Province reputedly viewed their auspicious lion dance as a covert form of anti-Qing resistance (Slovenz-Low 1994: 189–191). Folklore suggests that lion dance performances were a means of fundraising, recruiting, and undercover messaging for anti-Qing revolutionaries, while lion dance training was a way of practising martial arts without arousing suspicion from Qing officials. This agenda may have been true in some cases, but as I discussed earlier, the average kung fu group in Southern China was not actively involved in full-blown sedition. Instead, a stance of resistance infused martial practices with meaning and value.

[23] http://www.hongluck.ca/lion-dance-history.php accessed (30 August 2013).

An anti-Qing stance is integral to two of lion dance's key components. First is the name. Nineteenth-century kung fu practitioners thought of their animal mask costume as an "awakened lion" [*síng sī*, 醒獅], which is a term that persists today. Awakening the lion meant bringing it to life through kung fu stances and stepping, but it was also an allusion to awakening China. Starting with losses during the first Opium War (1839–1842), China experienced a "century of humiliation" [*baak nihn gwokchí*, 百年國恥] brought on by a series of unequal treaties with Western nations and imperial Japan (Scott 2008: 2–3). The vigorous martial sound and movement of the awakened lion was an aspirational metaphor, symbolically calling on China to throw off not only the Manchurian Qing Dynasty, but also the foreign powers intent on carving up the country (Liu 1981: 85–86).

To this day, kung fu clubs ritually "awaken" their lion masks before use. To begin, two lion dancers put on the costume, sit on the ground, and mime sleeping by closing the mask's eyes. Then, the head instructor or another senior member "dots the eyes" [*dím jīng*, 點睛], which includes tying a red ribbon on the lion's horn before marking the lion's eyes, horn, mouth, and tail with a paintbrush dipped in liquid cinnabar. A carved piece of ginger contains the red fluid, and a senior member explained to me that the ginger represents the Earth because it is a root, while cinnabar represents Heaven because of its auspicious red colour and association with immortality in Chinese alchemy. Other members told me that either the red ribbon was practical because it lets dancers know which masks are awake and which ones are not yet ready to use, or it symbolized "taming" the lion by binding it. At Hong Luck, I observed that Master Paul recited rhyming couplets invoking the lion's spirit as he dotted the eyes, while Master Jim performed the procedure in silence. After the eye dotting, the gong and drum ensemble plays, leading the lion in a brief performance to complete the awakening.

The second persistent anti-Qing lion dance symbol is the climax of the ritual action. The highlight of a typical performance has long been when the lion "eats" a bunch of vegetables, then spit them back out. This sequence, called "plucking-the-greens" [*chói chēng*, 採青], is a series of double entendre. In Cantonese, both the verb "to pluck" [*chói*, 採] and the noun "vegetable" [*choi*, 菜] sound like "good fortune" [*chòih*, 財], so a lion plucking a vegetable, and then spitting it back out in many pieces, signifies multiplication of wealth. The Cantonese word for "green" [*chēng*, 青] used in the name plucking-the-greens, however, is homophonous with the name of the Qing Dynasty [*Chīng*, 清], so the lion is symbolically eating the historical oppressors. Traditionally, a lucky red envelope containing money is tied to the vegetable, which lion dancers would keep when they spat out the broken-up greens. The plucking-the-greens sequence remains universal in Southern Chinese lion dance traditions and is an essential part of contemporary performances. It was—and is—an important source of income for kung fu groups, whether that is to support revolutionary aspirations or just to keep the lights on in the training hall.

Lion dance's long history has led to many regional variants flourishing in today's world, both within China and in other parts of Asia. In China, there is a basic bifurcation between Northern and Southern styles. In the North, lion costumes look somewhat more realistic than in the South, and Northern dancing tends to be both more acrobatic and more feline. Hong Luck's lion dancing is a typical example of the Southern style, demonstrating powerful movements grounded in kung fu, as well as a fantastical costume that observers in Toronto often mistook for a "dragon."[24] Within the broader Chinese world, there is also a green, flat-faced, Hokkien lion in Fujian Province and Taiwan, as well as a related masked dance among the Hakka people of Guangdong and Fujian that uses a "unicorn" instead of a lion.[25] From an organological perspective, the percussion used in the various types of Chinese lion dance is similar to the ensembles used in Chinese religion, ritual, and opera, though the exact sizes, shapes, and types vary (Jones 1995: 104). Other Asian nations have lion dance as well, such as Japan, Korea, and Indonesia, albeit with divergent musical accompaniment that includes melodic instruments as well as pitched percussion.

In Southern China and the Chinese diaspora, Southern lion dance predominates, with subdivisions into traditional and contemporary variants. The style associated with traditional kung fu clubs like Hong Luck is Futsan [*Fahtsāan*, 佛山], referring to the Foshan area of Guangdong Province. The contemporary style associated with lion dance competitions is Hoksan [*Hohksāan*, 鶴山], which refers to the Heshan region of Guangdong. Both Futsan and Hoksan troupes perform the plucking-the-greens sequence and

---

[24] Lion dancing uses a mask costume animated by two people, while "dragon dancing" [*móuh lùhng*, 舞龍] uses a puppet on poles manipulated by a group of people. The biggest dragons can require as much as a hundred performers. Interestingly, the dragon dances I have observed in Toronto and Hong Kong utilized the same instruments and rhythms as Southern Chinese lion dancing.

[25] "Unicorn dancing" [*móuh kèihlèuhn*, 舞麒麟] is based on a mythical creature that, like the Southern Chinese lion, has little resemblance to any natural animal. Hakka people are a Han Chinese group now found primarily in Southern China, but whose origins lie farther north thanks to a series of migrations over the last two millennia. Their name literally means "guest family" [*Haakgā*, 客家].

use the same percussion ensemble (with slightly different rhythms),[26] but their lions differ in appearance and movement style. Generally speaking, Futsan movements are rooted in martial arts, with deep stances and powerful action, while Hoksan movements are more catlike and acrobatic. In a world of air travel, global commerce, and internet access, there has been increasing amounts of mutual exposure and cross-pollination, so these categories have started to break down. As a result, many groups use a hybrid Fut-Hok style of costume and movement. To make matters more complicated, there are still some Hoksan groups who use a more traditional, kung fu–based style, as well as Futsan groups that perform with more contemporary, acrobatic flair. Broadly speaking, however, Futsan and Hoksan are the older and newer schools, respectively.

Visually, all Southern Chinese lions share a family resemblance—with a few significant differences. Futsan lions have a curved mouth and a pointy horn, while Hoksan lions have a straight mouth and a rounded horn. Traditionally, Southern lion costumes of both varieties used a big head (covering the dancer's whole torso) and long tail (approximately three metres or almost ten feet), while contemporary designs have moved towards smaller heads (covering just the dancer's upper torso) and shorter tails (approximately two metres or six-and-a-half feet). Both traditional and modernized lions are available from various manufacturers and retailers, but the global trend is towards a more contemporary style for both Futsan and Hoksan lion costumes.

Traditional kung fu lions are meant to look tough and fearsome, with big heads and long tails that take up a lot of space. The beard, eyebrows, and eyelashes are bristling, crimped, or stringy, while the fur used to accent other parts of the head and body is short and sparse. There are three main colour schemes, symbolizing the three sworn brothers from the aforementioned *Romance of the Three Kingdoms* (see Figure 2.3). I have already introduced Guan Yu; his comrades at arms are Liu Bei [*Làuh Beih*, 劉備], the elder leader of the trio, and Zhang Fei [*Jēung Fēi*, 張飛], the youngest and most pugnacious of the group. A Zhang Fei lion is the most aggressive, which it suitable for a new kung fu club and/or one that is ready to fight. The beard is short, and the colour scheme uses black fur with green or white accents on the head and body. In Hong Luck's early days, they often used a Zhang Fei lion head for parades. Guan Yu is loyal, righteous, and brave, so his lion is

---

[26] Hong Luck drummers have picked up some Hoksan rhythms, but their use in performance has sometimes been the target of censure. I will discuss these rhythms and the issues surrounding them in the next chapter.

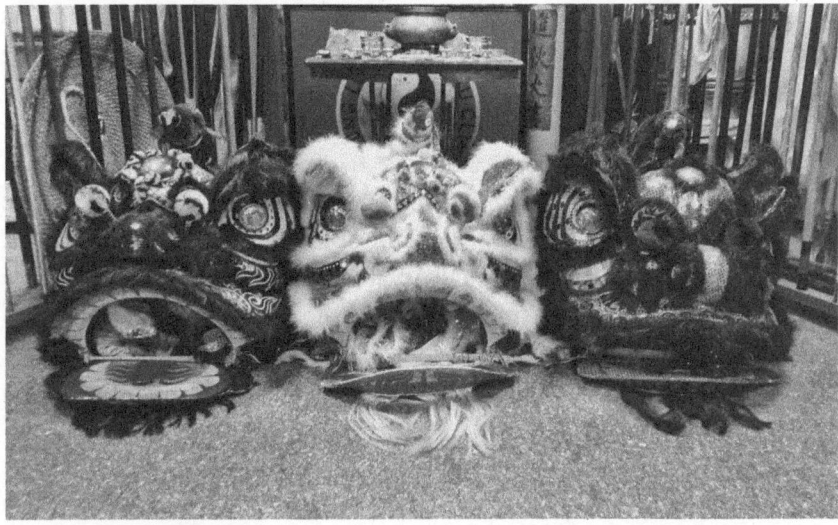

Figure 2.3 Futsan lion heads
Credits: Colin P. McGuire

suitable for any kung fu club. His medium-bearded lion has black fur with a red face and black alternating with red for the body. Liu Bei's lion is noble and auspicious. It has white fur, a long beard, and a multi-coloured body that uses the colours associated with the five elements: black, white, yellow, red, and green. A Liu Bei lion is suitable for an established kung fu club with an older master, though other clubs use them because of their auspicious appearance. During my fieldwork, most of Hong Luck's lions were in the Guan Yu or Liu Bei styles. They had large heads and long tails that were marginally smaller/shorter than in previous generations, but not fully reduced to contemporary proportions.

The advent of lion dance competitions in Singapore drove changes in both performance and construction, making lions lighter, more agile, and better able to perform acrobatic stunts. According to the now-defunct *History of Singapore Dragon and Lion Dance* website formerly maintained by Singapore's National Heritage Board (last updated 2013), 1967 marked the country's first National Pugilistic Competition, which naturally included lion dance. Despite being more numerous, Southern lion dancers could not compete against the flashy moves of the lone Northern lion dance troupe. Thereafter, Hoksan innovators adapted their style to become "Southern lion Northern dance" [*Làahm sī Bāk móuh*, 南獅北舞], emphasizing feline movement and spectacular jumps on various types of apparatus. As competitions became larger and more international, the crowd-pleasing Hoksan lion dance spread around the world. Top competitors no longer need to practise martial arts at all because the foundation of the movement has changed; instead, they typically specialize exclusively in lion dance, although some martial arts groups still compete at a high level. In addition to reducing the size, length, and weight of the lion to accommodate acrobatics, competition lions began to come in an array of bright colours, with body and head trimmed in luxuriant strips of fur. Some contemporary heads now incorporate holographic paper into their designs, or even LED lights. The pleasant colours, fuzziness, and bright accents give them a friendly or even cute appearance.

Hong Luck has been resistant to lion dance trends but has nonetheless made slow changes over time. As I mentioned earlier, the club's Futsan lions had become smaller and lighter over time, and they even had a pair of smallish Hoksan heads (although they still danced Futsan style while using them). Towards the end of my fieldwork, Hong Luck also started using a couple new colour schemes. In the fall of 2015, the president of Hong Luck's tong association summoned me to help him collect a pair of new lion heads that were gifts from the PRC's consulate in Toronto. Upon arrival, a functionary presented us with a selection of contemporary Futsan lion heads in a rainbow of colours. The president and I, along with two other senior members, quickly discovered that there were no lions in the colour schemes of the three sworn brothers. We agreed that pink, orange, blue, and green lions did not behoove Hong Luck's kung fu ethos, and so we chose a yellow/gold lion with red highlights and a red lion with gold/yellow highlights. These are the two colours in the flag of the PRC and figure prominently in festive decorations for Chinese New Year because of their auspicious associations with happiness, wealth, and good fortune. This negotiation of symbolism shows a stance on lion dancing that privileges its meanings. A bright blue lion might have been eye-catching, but it would have been lacking in visual qualities contributing to its value as a ritual.

Everybody at Hong Luck was aware of the flashy moves found in the Hoksan style, but there was a generational division of opinion about it. The younger lion dancers had no problem with practising Hoksan jumps where the person playing the head would leap while the person in the tail would propel their partner into the air by grabbing onto their belt. Both my lion dance teachers were in their early twenties, and they had no reservations about teaching us students to do jumps. One evening, however, Master Paul Chan dropped into the lion dance class to give us some pointers ahead of our performance at the upcoming wedding of one of his family members. He told us jumps were dangerous and far less important than demonstrating powerful stances, bringing the lion to life, and respecting ritual propriety. Furthermore, Master Paul also emphasized synchronizing the lion's action with the beats as central to the performance's coherence.

Although I practised jumping lion regularly throughout my time at Hong Luck, we rarely did jumps in public. The club's conservative stance, as explained by Master Paul, was an important factor in this dichotomy between private practice versus public performance. On the other hand, it was sometimes an issue of human resources. Performing jumps requires well-matched partners because the tail performer needs to be strong enough to lift and even carry the person in the head. There also needs to be good coordination between the partners, so it helps if they practice together regularly. Often, people who knew how to lion dance but did not attend the weekly class would still help with Hong Luck's lion dance gigs, in which case it was easier and safer to stick with basic choreography. Nonetheless, there was some debate around the club about needing to compete with other kung fu clubs in Toronto who either performed in a hybrid Fut-Hok style or had jumped entirely on the Hoksan bandwagon. Hong Luck's long history and deep community roots helped the club continue to get gigs anyway, but during my fieldwork in Hong Kong, Master Joe Kwong [*Kwong Jóubóu Sīfú*, 鄺組寶師傅] of the New Asia Kung Fu Club told me that his group would not be doing many lion dance performances if they only did traditional Futsan style. He had to hybridize—or forgo that income stream.

Historical Context of Chinese Martial Sound

I introduced some of the ancient connections between music and martial arts in the Prologue of this book, which I will now revisit. There is historical precedent for thinking of kung fu percussion as martial sound, which contextualizes my consultants' comments about their drumming not being music, per se. In Sun Tzu's previously mentioned discussion of gongs and drums from the sixth-century BCE military treatise *The Art of War*, it is notable that the Chinese text (see Wing 1988: 98) does not contain the characters for "music" [*yāmngohk*, 音樂] in this section. Instead, the text simply uses the names of the instruments, "gong" [*lòh*, 鑼] and "drum" [*gú*, 鼓]. Sun Tzu proposed that what I call martial sound organizes troop movements and rouses the energy of soldiers. He further claimed that it could be used offensively to "take away the heart of their generals," and an ancient commentator on that passage of the text clarified that thunderous percussion would "startle their perceptions and make them fear your awesome martial power" (trans. Cleary 2003: 125). Master Sun's stance on gongs and drums was unmistakeably bellicose and strategic, completely lacking in consideration for "musical" niceties.

As for "real" music, a venerable Chinese encyclopaedia compiled circa 239 BCE titled *Master Lü's Spring and Autumn Annals* [*Léuihsih Chēun Chāu*, 《呂氏春秋》] defined it as "the harmony between Heaven and Earth, and the perfect blend of Yin and Yang" (trans. Knoblock and Riegel 2000: 138). The Annals go on to circumscribe music's function as a ceremonial procedure that was both product and producer of cosmic order, emphasizing musicking as an essential form of ritual propriety. The text mentions powerful drumming, but it suggests that such sounds are best kept separate from music because "the more extravagant the music, the gloomier are the people, the more disordered the state, and the more debased its ruler" (trans. Knoblock and Riegel 2000: 140). This does not mean that heavy percussion was forbidden, but rather that it was restricted in its function and use. More specifically, the Annals suggest that "[i]f these sounds (percussion) are employed to shock the mental energies, startle the ears and eyes, and agitate the inborn nature, it is permissible" (trans. Knoblock and Riegel 2000: 140). Here we see that martial sound would definitely have had a place on the battlefield or in exorcisms, but not in music.

Distinctions between different forms of humanly organized sound have had an ongoing place in Chinese aesthetics, reflecting larger systems of cultural coherence. Within the category of music-as-music, there is an important stylistic dichotomy of between "civil" [*màhn*, 文] and "martial" [*móuh*, 武] pieces, instruments, and genres (Jones 1995: 104). This binary is part of a Chinese world-view that divides, organizes, and interprets society according to "civil and martial" [*màhn móuh*, 文武] (Gawlikowski 1987). These spheres overlap and interpenetrate each other in a mutually constitutive balance embodied by the Taoist cosmological principle of "yin and yang," [*yàm yèuhng*, 陰陽], where existence is made up of equal opposites that are in a dynamic, every-changing, energetic interrelationship. The yin principle is quiet, soft, feminine, and so on, while yang is loud, hard, male, and so on. The martial principle has yin associations with death, chaos, and destruction, although it functions by means of yang qualities like strength, action, and bravery. This interpenetration is echoed in the civil principle, which is yang because it focuses on order, growth, and prosperity, although its virtues include yin qualities like peace, gentleness, and artistic refinement. Ultimately, civil and martial are coextensive and mutually generative because civil order is forged with martial vigour, while martial strength becomes virtuous through civil discipline. Southern Chinese kung fu and lion dance percussion may involve musicking, but it is so far to one pole of the civil and martial principle that it exceeds the category of music to become martial sound.

Discussion and Summary

The Hong Luck Kung Fu Club's blurred genre of martial arts is like a rope plaited from many separate strands; it is more than the sum of the individual threads. In this chapter, I have parsed Southern Shaolin martial arts in general, the Choi Lee Fut and Do Pi styles in specific, the Tang Dynasty courtly lion dance, kung fu lion dancing from the Qing Dynasty, contemporary lion dance competition, and Chinese socio-cultural aesthetics of civil and martial in musicking. I have also discussed the efforts of the Republican-era Nationalist government and Chinese martial arts reformers to modernize kung fu. Although discourses of rational self-strengthening might not have the same appeal as myths about Shaolin warrior monks and anti-Qing revolutionaries, the spirit of the post-Qing kung fu reformation has had a profound impact on Chinese martial arts that deserves greater acknowledgment from the community of practice. In separating out these strands, my aim has been to show the rich palimpsest of historical models that undergird Hong Luck's superscribed practices. As I summarize, I would like to reemphasize that Hong Luck's kung fu does not actually separate martial arts from lion dance or drumming, but rather makes them all in the same mould.

In this chapter I have also given a brief history of Chinese experiences in Canada, including the founding of Hong Luck, to contextualize the Cantonese traditions that I encountered during my fieldwork. The stories and histories of resistance in kung fu and lion dance undergird Hong Luck's ethos of empowerment. Hand-to-hand warfare has long been obsolete on the battlefield, and yet archaic hand combat skills embody the ideal of self-defence. Notwithstanding the invincibility of kung fu in films, neither anti-Qing martial artists in China nor Hong Luck's founders in Canada were likely to literally fight the system using their kung fu. Nonetheless, martial arts played an important role in both situations. In nineteenth-century Guangdong, kung fu and lion dance were ways of fomenting revolution, or at least maintaining a spirit of resistance. In Hong Luck's early days, self-defence skills allowed members to act against racial violence in their neighbourhood, but, more broadly, their strong and steadfast presence in Chinatown provided heroic inspiration for their community. Kung fu was also a tool for diplomacy, outreach, and mutual understanding, building bridges with non-Chinese Canadians through both public performance and by teaching to people of all ethnic backgrounds.

The woke kung fu lion remains a potent symbol of Chinese strength, and many of Hong Luck's masks still have the Chinese characters for "awakened lion" [síng sī, 醒獅] painted on them. In the club's early days, they would often use the green/black, Zhang Fei, fighting lion for parades and public performances. China was still asleep, caught in the nightmare of the Cultural Revolution (1966–1976), while Hong Luck was wakeful, asserting Chinese Canadian power and presence in Toronto's Chinatown. China is now a superpower with both political and economic clout; the metaphorical lion is awake and roaring. Chinese Canadians are no longer subject to the systemic discrimination of yore, though Hong Luck members still reported cases of interpersonal racism towards them. On 22 June 2006, then–Prime Minister Stephen Harper offered a full apology for the exclusion of, and discrimination against, the Chinese in Canada, with an emphasis on the injustice of the Head Tax. He also recognized the key part played by the Chinese railway workers in Canada's confederation as a country. With the rise of China on the global scene and the much-improved position of Chinese Canadians, resistance to domination is no longer as essential as it once was, but empowering narratives continue to inspire new generations of practitioners.

There remains more to Hong Luck than martial arts. The club has continued to provide a familiar social space to the elders as a tong. Their children and grandchildren, as well as those of other Chinese Canadian families, train at the club to learn about the culture of their ancestors. In addition to kung fu classes, Hong Luck has also sometimes offered Chinese language training and "calligraphy" [syūfaat, 書法] workshops. As Uncle Poi told me, an important part of the club's mandate has been to promote cultural understanding. Lion dancing and percussion are the most public expressions of

Hong Luck's kung fu, continuing to preserve and promote Cantonese culture in Toronto. Through these various activities, the club has offered naturalized Chinese Canadians, Canadian-born Chinese, and non-Chinese people a way of participating in the Chinatown community.

The Hong Luck Kung Fu Club continues to serve the tong associations and the Chinatown community, but the scene is changing. Competition for lion dance gigs is increasing because there are now over ten kung fu clubs in the Greater Toronto Area with active troupes. A new generation of potential students is likely to eschew Hong Luck's traditions for the showy acrobatics of contemporary Hoksan lion dancing or the perceived effectiveness of modern combat sports like mixed martial arts (MMA). The death of Master Paul Chan in 2012 caused much sorrow, but it also fostered discussion about the future direction of the club. When Master Jim Chan took over as Hong Luck's head instructor, training returned to the status quo. Sadly, Master Jim also passed away shortly after I left Toronto in the fall of 2016. For now, being a not-for-profit and having ownership of the building are the club's saving graces as it pursues a highly traditional agenda in an increasingly modern world. Nonetheless, many members have expressed their concern about Hong Luck's future, which is a subject I return to in this book's conclusion.

3

Layered Meanings of Lion Dance

Introduction

This chapter focuses on lion dance with percussion accompaniment, which is the most public showcase of the Hong Luck Kung Fu Club's blurred genre. With deep roots in ritual exorcism and blessing, lion dancing is also a performance of identity, a form of martial display, and an entertaining cultural spectacle, resulting in multivalent meanings. In Toronto, the diasporic, multicultural, and multigenerational context contributes to the lion dance's potential for heterogeneous-yet-coextensive significances. I summarized some of the main symbols associated with lion dance, kung fu, and their martial sound in the previous chapter. Semiotically, those are general signs that achieve meaning through the conventions of linguistic definition based on rational cognitive processes (Turino 2014 further to Peirce 1985 [1903]). This chapter continues to engage with symbolism but moves beyond common conventions to provide thicker description. I also present more ethnographic research data, which is based on the commentary of my consultants and informed by my participant-observer experience as a lion dancer.

During my fieldwork, lion dance parades were Hong Luck's largest public activity, which is why I have chosen to focus much of this chapter on ethnography of Chinese New Year celebrations.[1] Kung fu demonstrations with percussion accompaniment were much less frequent and will be reserved for later chapters. The description, explanation, and interpretation in this chapter stem from my participation in seventeen lion dance parades and

---

[1] The Hong Luck Kung Fu Club usually does two lion dance processions per year in Toronto's Spadina/Dundas Chinatown. Most of the discussion in this chapter is focused on the Lunar New Year parade because of the importance of that festive celebration in Chinese culture. The overall sequence, organization, and ritual action are basically the same for both processions. The Hong Luck anniversary lion dance parade in August usually has more members participating than the Chinese New Year procession because the weather is warmer and people have fewer obligations in the summer, but also because it engenders a sense of group loyalty. There is less participation in Hong Luck's anniversary parade from Chinatown's patrons, however, due to the lion dance ritual being more associated with New Years.

Martial Sound. Colin P. McGuire, Oxford University Press. © Oxford University Press 2024.
DOI: 10.1093/oso/9780197775936.003.0003

over eighty lion dance performances, during a period of approximately eight years (2008–2016). In Toronto, this included working with Hong Luck, as well as other local kung fu groups founded by senior students who became teachers in their own rights but still maintained their ties with the club and its founders. My acceptance as a researcher at Hong Luck was contingent on my ongoing participation in their martial arts, dance, and musicking. As a result, I have a lion's-eye view of their practices because, by my fifth year of fieldwork, I ended up with the privilege and responsibility of being the most regular lion dance performer at the club. The flip side of this situation is that I spent relatively less time on the outside looking in at performances than I have being right in the middle of them. In addition, I have also studied private archival videos from Hong Luck, as well as recordings of events in which I participated. Through performance, my teachers had regular opportunities to shape my embodied knowledge by intersubjectively evaluating, critiquing, and thereby informing future performances. Their collective and individual views of lion dance, kung fu, and martial sound have thus been integral to my research and undergird my interpretation. New Years' parades were particularly important for getting this feedback because a much larger range of Hong Luck members attended, including elders and seniors who were no longer active in regular performances or weekly classes.

In general, I discuss lion dance as a ritual, albeit one whose complex cultural and performative roles thwart simple categorization. I begin with an overview of lion dance parades, including a description of the movement and sound, followed by a discussion of people's negotiation of the ritual sequence and repertoire of rhythms. Next, I provide an interpretation of lion dance as a performance with important implications for people's sense of self—even when the ceremonial aspects of the ritual are downplayed. Then, I discuss how lion dance and martial sound work to construct Chinatown's space as a diasporic community in an urban multicultural place. First, however, I position my discussion in relation to existing studies of lion dance, as well as theories of ritual and performance ethnography.

Lion Dance Scholarship, Notation, and Ritual

There is a growing body of scholarship on lion dance that has cleared a path for my own work by establishing a foundation of knowledge on the subject. The most internationally well-known style is the Southern (a.k.a., Cantonese) lion dance, which has received a majority of attention in print. The dominant approach has been to focus on lion dance's symbolism, costuming, historical roots, and ritual functions (Feltham 2009; Hu 1995; Kim 1975; Liu 1981; Yap 2017). While Cantonese lion dancing belongs to an ancient cultural heritage of masked dances, its direct origins lie in the nineteenth century with kung fu practitioners in Guangdong Province. A major factor in the lion dance's endurance as a symbol of identity is its link to martial arts and strength; it has acted as a public expression of fighting spirit in the face of oppression. This form of symbolic resistance is empowering, and it has extended from the secret societies who positioned themselves against a Manchu-controlled Qing Dynasty, through to the discrimination and segregation faced by Chinese people overseas. While many scholars recognize the connections of Southern Chinese lion dance to kung fu, none have discussed lion dancing from a martial arts perspective, which is a gap that I aim to fill.

Patrons most often commission traditional Southern Chinese lion dances to perform a para-liturgical function that anthropologist Heleanor Feltham has summed up as the protection of liminal spaces, times, and transitions (2009: 111). Typical examples include New Years, store openings, and weddings. The loud percussion acts as the lion's roar, and, combined with the fearsome aspect of the costume, this martial sound dispels what Hong Luck elders call "nefarious energy" [chèh hei, 邪氣], paving the way for good fortune. As I described in the previous chapter, the climax of the performance is when the lion finds, "eats," and vigorously spits out a leafy green vegetable. The plucking-the-greens sequence and the physical appearance of the costume itself are central to typical explanations of the symbols that make up lion dance's ritual meaning. Edward Schiefflin (1985), however, has criticized such conventionalized approaches to ritual in general because they belie the significance of performance, participation, and individual stances on the generation of meaning. Similarly, Victor Turner (1977) has suggested that ethnographers should focus on the dynamic processes of ritual, rather than reifying the product.

Some scholars have engaged with lion dance performance in more ethnographic ways, particularly in diasporic contexts. Most notably, performance-studies scholar Madeline Slovenz has written richly detailed accounts of lion dancing in a New York City kung fu club, looking at everything from training and pre-performance preparation to parades and post-performance activities (Slovenz 1987; Slovenz-Low 1994). Her work focuses more on description than interpretation, perhaps because Slovenz's research involved more observation than participation. Her consultants only allowed her to play the role of the "big head Buddha" [*daaih tàuh faht*, 大頭佛], a masked character that sometimes accompanies lion dance, but she did not do any lion dancing or play the instruments.[2] One must wonder why Slovenz did not discuss gender roles in lion dance, because she could not have been unaware of the traditional exclusion of women. I flag this issue now, but I am reserving a discussion of gender for the next chapter. Ethnographic studies of other diasporic Chinese communities have engaged with how lion dance has shifted from being an imported, regional, ritual practice of first-generation Cantonese migrants, to becoming a pan-Chinese, multivocal, cultural performance of diverse identities with participants including second (and higher) generations away from Southern China, as well as people with roots in non-Cantonese parts of Greater China and even non-Chinese (Li 2017; Wu 2015).

Educational perspectives on lion dance have often focused on identity and culture, though approaches have varied. Music scholar Henry Johnson (2005) has looked at the way a lion dance group hosted by a New Zealand secondary school provided opportunities for Chinese students both to perform their ethno-cultural identity and to form it through participation in lion dance. Similarly, education scholar Chan Mei Hsiu (2001) tailored a crash course in lion dance to quickly teach various aspects of heritage culture to a group of Chinese American students. Finally, Patricia Shehan Campbell and Han Kuo-Huang (1996) wrote a small workbook for Chinese percussion ensembles that uses Western music notation to teach simple rhythm pieces, including the lion dance. Unfortunately, they only represent the costume and movement with text and still images, so the dance itself is conspicuous by its absence. There are also some problems with the way Western notation implies rhythmic concepts that are foreign to the practice, but the book is intended as a pedagogical tool, not a scholarly treatise.

English-language texts have presented useful information about lion dancing but little detail about the accompanying percussion, whereas some

---

[2] During her fieldwork, Slovenz trained in kung fu with a New York–based master from Guangdong named Chan Taisan [*Chàhn Taisāan Sīfú*, 陳泰山師傅] but did not learn lion dance from him. Showing how small the world can be, Chan Taisan also taught at Hong Luck when he lived in Toronto for a time.

Chinese-language books have provided transcriptions of drum patterns (Li and Liu 1985; Liang 2008). These examples notate dance separately from percussion, and both are fairly skeletal. These texts also tend towards prescription and a somewhat laudatory tone. An article by Liu Chang-lin (2011) gives a more in-depth transcription of modern lion dance drumming and helpfully adds the names of the choreography on top of the notation. Unfortunately for readers only familiar with Western notation, however, the transcription uses Chinese ciphers. A partial solution lies with Zhang Boyu from the Central Conservatory of Music in Beijing, who has proposed a hybrid notation for the study of Ten Variations Gong and Drum [*Sahpfān Lòhgú*, 十番鑼鼓] music from Jiangsu Province (1997: 25–29).[3] The salient features of his approach are the incorporation of vocables that practitioners use to speak the "gong and drum text" [*lòhgú gīng*, 鑼鼓經] and the lack of time signatures, both of which are designed to respect the organization of this type of percussion music into phrases, rather than forcing it into Western meter. Zhang still uses the symbols from Western staff notation, which makes it easy to read by anyone trained in that system.

Building on the approaches of other scholars studying Chinese percussion, my transcriptions in this chapter (and elsewhere in the book) use modified Western notation that incorporates vocables and/or choreography, as appropriate. This type of transcription is also inspired by the work of other scholars who include more than just sound in their notation, such as Regula Qureshi's (1986) charts of performer-audience interaction in the performance of qawwali music. While I hope that my transcriptions will prove a useful supplement for readers, I am also respecting the limits set by my consultants: they would not permit me to transcribe whole routines or to attempt a thorough catalogue of the personal variations performed by individual drummers. I have been granted permission to transcribe and share an example of the mini performances that occur during public parades (e.g., Chinese New Year), which contain all of the essential features of a lion dance.

Victor Turner has defined ritual as "a stereotyped sequence of activities involving gestures, words, and objects, performed in a sequestered place, and designed to influence preternatural entities or forces on behalf of the actors' goals and interests" (1973: 1100). While this description works for some

---

[3] Some readers may be familiar with the Mandarin name for Ten Variations Gong and Drum: *Shífān Luógǔ*.

of Hong Luck's lion dancing, in other situations the supernatural aspect is secondary to (re)affirming social bonds, (re)constructing cultural identity, and/or (re)creating the space of Chinatown. In fact, it is not uncommon for there to be negotiation between patrons and performers, as well as internally among Hong Luck elders, seniors, and juniors, regarding the relative importance of the lion dance's various functions and how these should be manifested. Differences of opinion are in line with performance-studies scholar Richard Schechner's observation that "rituals are not safe deposit vaults of accepted ideas but in many cases dynamic performative systems generating new materials and recombining traditional actions in new ways" (1993: 228).

It is useful to separate lion dance functions for analytical purposes, but I would like to emphasize that they are not mutually exclusive. Depending on the perspectives of performers, patrons, and audiences, various meanings are possible simultaneously and/or sequentially. For all forms of performance, Schechner proposes that the seeming opposition of ritual efficacy and theatrical entertainment are actually the poles of a continuum where "[n]o performance is pure efficacy or pure entertainment" (1974: 468). The overlapping gradient scale of entertainment/efficacy has proven a fruitful interpretive frame for Timothy Cooley's (2006) work on folklore festivals as rituals of identity in Poland, showing that the model applies far beyond theatre. I thus position lion dance as mystical and social, practical and performative. The degree of efficacy versus entertainment that people experience differs according to context and viewpoint, resulting in multiple, non-contradictory stances for participants.

In order to engage with lion dance as a lived experience, I focus on the way it is presented by Hong Luck, which will be similar to many diasporic Chinese martial arts groups. My discussion of this ritual performance practice is rooted in an analysis of the signification process, privileging context, performance, event, and situation as being key determinants of ritual meaning (Turner 1975: 150–151). By moving past normative ritual symbolism, I am engaging with the fluidity of meaning creation where:

(1) every musical sound, performance or dance movement, and contextual feature that affects an actual perceiver is a sign, and (2) every perceiver is affected by signs in relation to his or her own personal history of experience, which is at once a partially unique but largely shared social experience. (Turino 2014: 188)

Organization of Lion Dance Parades

New Years is the most important holiday on the Chinese calendar, and Southern lion dance is an important part of the celebrations in Cantonese Guangdong, Guangxi, Hong Kong, Macau, and their associated diaspora. The traditional Chinese calendar is lunar, so the festivities occur at a different time every year relative to the (now) internationally used Gregorian solar calendar. The first day of Chinese New Year typically falls around the end of January or beginning of February, though celebrations lasts for several weeks on either side of the actual day. In China, this whole period is a civic holiday. It is not a holiday in Canada, so Hong Luck's lion dance parades were usually scheduled on the next weekend after the first day of the New Year—never before, which would be inauspicious. In Chinese, New Years is often called the Spring Festival [*Chēun Jit*, 春節], but in Toronto the northerly latitude means that the festivities usually fall in the dead of winter.[4]

As compared to some of Toronto's other parades, such as the large-scale Santa Claus Parade and Saint Patrick's Day Parade, Hong Luck's Chinese New Year lion dance processions require active participation from audiences as patrons. The parades do not occur on blocked-off streets thronged by spectators more or less passively watching. Instead, they happen right on the sidewalks, making stops to perform for patrons. That being said, Hong Luck has also sometimes participated in more presentational events, such as Canada Day parades organized by the National Congress of Chinese Canadians [*Chyùhn Gā Wàhyàhn Lyùhnwúi*, 全加華人聯會], or China Day parades organized by the PRC's consulate.

In the days leading up to a parade, Hong Luck representatives hand out flyers in Chinatown that announce the day and time that their lions will roam the streets (see Figure 3.1). These red paper leaflets are written in (mostly) traditional Chinese characters that go from right to left in vertically descending columns, which signifies several things. Left-to-right horizontal rows of text are now more common than the old-style, right-to-left vertical columns. Hong Luck's notices therefore show the club's stance on tradition, acting as an immediate sign to literate Sinophones through visual layout. Furthermore, the use of traditional characters adds another layer to the stance on tradition. The PRC has promoted simplified Chinese

---

[4] Another name for Chinese New Year is Agricultural Calendar New Year [*Nùhnglihk Sānnìhn*, 農曆新年].

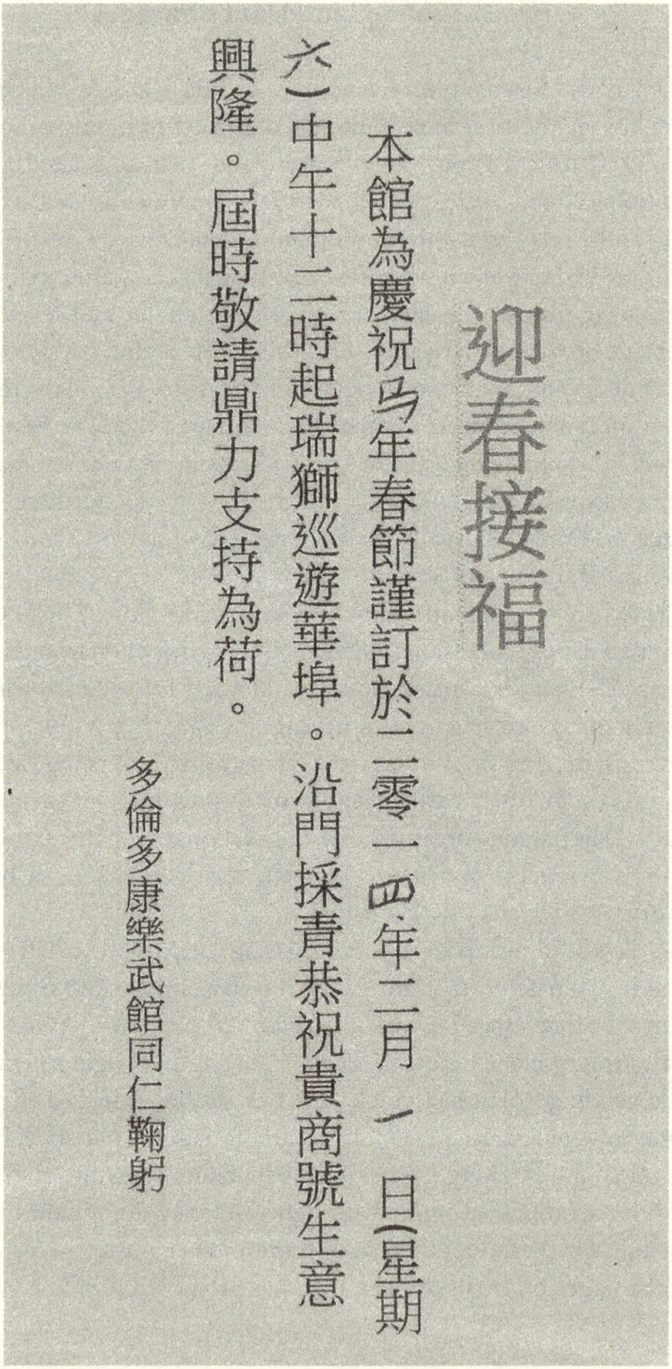

迎春接福

本館為慶祝马年春節謹訂於二零一四年二月 一 日(星期六)中午十二時起瑞獅巡遊華埠。沿門採青恭祝貴商號生意興隆。屆時敬請鼎力支持為荷。

多倫多康樂武館同仁鞠躬

Figure 3.1 Lion dance parade flyer, February 2014
Credits: Colin P. McGuire

characters since the 1950s, and these were later adopted by Singapore and Malaysia. A senior Hong Luck member told me that the club had tried using simplified characters for a while as a way of showing a stance on supporting the PRC but found too many people could not read them. Using traditional script is thus partly a question of intelligibility, because Hong Kong, Macau, Taiwan, and most of the diaspora have retained traditional characters. To further complicate the issue, some simplified characters were used during my fieldwork as widely understood shorthand or cursive variants, such as the simplified character for "horse" [*máh*, 马 instead of 馬] on the flyer in Figure 3.1.

The colour of the paper is as significant as the style of writing. Red is considered happy and auspicious in Chinese culture, so it is used for New Year's and wedding decorations as well as in the paper envelopes of lucky money that are given at these events.[5] Beyond this conventional symbolism, red also has an iconic resemblance to burning coals and fiery chili peppers, making it a warm colour. Consequently, Chinese New Year is fuelled by red decorations that signify not only happiness and luck, but also warmth. In Chinese, successful social events are literally "hot and noisy" [*yiht naauh*, 熱鬧], meaning bustling with people and filled with sound. Hong Luck's red flyers thus use colour to foreshadow the "heat" of a lion dance parade, which includes the noise of the gong and drum ensemble to complete the desirable hot and noisy atmosphere.

If one looks more closely at these lion dance notices, the style of language also gives clues about what audiences can expect and how to participate. They are written in a formal and polite manner, which suggests ritual propriety. The text explains that those whose doorways are prepared for the auspicious lion to pluck the greens will be wished good luck, success, and prosperous commerce. Hong Luck seniors emphasized the importance of this blessing to all new lion dancers because, for some members of the local community, commercial success in the coming year depended on the New Year's lion dance. The flyers do not explicitly say how to prepare the doorway, so recipients are expected to have the required cultural knowledge—not to mention Chinese literacy. At the same time, I observed

---

[5] Traditional Chinese wedding gowns are red, though many Canadian-born Chinese opt for a white gown. It is not unusual for Cantonese brides to have a wardrobe change at some point during the day of their nuptials, which I observed when I attended a kung fu classmate's wedding. The double-wedding-dress system is also gaining popularity in Hong Kong, as attested by my Cantonese language teachers at CUHK.

that some non-Chinese patrons in Chinatown were still eager to participate, requiring on-the-spot coaching from Hong Luck members during parades.

With or without veggies, a "red packet" [*hùhng bāau*, 紅包] hung at the doorway signals that a patron wants a lion dance. As previously described, the crimson envelope contains money to pay for the performance. Chinese New Year is ostensibly about auspicating the earth's next trip around the sun, but it is more importantly a time for family and friends, which includes the important custom of older people giving small red packets stuffed with "lucky money" [*laihsih*, 利是] to the young and/or unmarried. Similarly, Hong Luck's lions go around Chinatown collecting the crimson envelopes of cash from shops, restaurants, and associations who are connected to the club through the network of mutual-aid groups or social ties. Other supporters have no affiliation but are willing to pay for the ritual exorcism blessing of a lion dance. There are also patrons who enjoy the entertaining spectacle for its own sake, without concern for any supernatural function, but they must still offer red packets to Hong Luck's lions. During eight years of fieldwork, I never collected an envelope with coins, so the minimum donation was five Canadian dollars. Some businesses had particularly strong ties to the club or deep concerns about ritual efficacy and gave as much as a couple hundred dollars, typically spread among several red packets. Notably, the more envelopes given, the longer the performance lasts because Hong Luck's lion dancers know to take their time when a patron is being generous.

During my fieldwork, not every business or association in Chinatown participated for various reasons. Sometimes it was simply a matter of timing and location. Some shops, offices, and tongs were closed at the time of the parade, although we once did a performance for a store that was not open but whose proprietor had left a lettuce and red packet hanging above their doorway. Some premises were above street level and were less likely to get a lion dance, even though Hong Luck's troupe would haul all their gear up several flights of stairs if necessary. In 2013, the owner of a Chinese bakery told me she was not interested in lion dancing because she was Christian and felt the ritual was just a superstition. Thereafter, Hong Luck stopped offering lion dances to this shop. Some shopkeepers and restauranteurs from Northern China did not get lion dances because it was an unfamiliar tradition from another part of China, although over time I observed some such people start to participate. For example, during the 2016 Chinese New Year parade, a Mandarin-speaking restaurant owner actually chased Hong Luck's troupe down the street after we passed her by. In previous years, she had not wanted a lion dance, but that year she exclaimed, "I'm part of Chinatown, too!" Her change of heart revealed her stance on the ritual's ability to construct the being of the neighbourhood; by participating, she expressed her belonging in the community through a tradition not her own. Some Mandarin speakers were more recalcitrant, however, and in 2013 the manager of a dumpling restaurant scolded me for offering a lion dance on behalf of Hong Luck. She angrily accused me of begging for money and shooed me out the door. Her reactions emphasized that some people in Chinatown not only were uninterested in lion dancing, but actively took a negative stance on the tradition.

Overview of Lion Dance Parades

The Hong Luck Kung Fu Club's Chinese New Year parades were quite consistent in their overall structure, which I observed through participation in 2009 to 2011, missed in 2012 because I was on exchange in Hong Kong (though I observed several parades while I was there), and joined again at Hong Luck from 2013 to 2016. The processions started at the club around noon, followed a route shaped like the Chinese character "ten" [sahp, 十] covering about two blocks in each direction through Chinatown's main intersection (Spadina Avenue and Dundas Street West), and returned back to where they began. These lion dance parades consisted of a string of individual performances for patrons connected by periods of walking as Hong Luck's troupe circumambulated the neighbourhood. Notably, the martial sound remained continuous, acting as the sonic glue that bonded separate rituals into a single event.

I describe the basic parade routine in greater detail later in this section, but, for now, I will provide a normative lion dance sequence to show the structure of the ritual that is repeated for each patron. This basic pattern typically lasts only about one minute on parade, but my teacher David assured me that it contained all the essential components. Practically speaking, these lion dances are reduced to only the indispensable aspects because of the sheer volume of performances required during parades that last a full afternoon. Some patrons may request longer rituals, which can be up to five or ten minutes long, but these were exceptions during my fieldwork. Hong Luck typically reserves longer performances for weddings, banquets, and store openings, which could be as much as twenty minutes, including extensions and elaborations of the basic sequence, as well as additional choreography not seen during parades. The essential elements of a lion dance, as performed during the New Year's procession, are as follows:

1. Walking (approaching)
2. Three-bows (respectful greeting)
3. Head-up and three-rises (dispersing negative energy)
4. Eating (testing, plucking, swallowing, and spitting)
5. Three-bows (respectful farewell)
6. Walking (leaving)

Most of Hong Luck's parades were between four and five hours long, which was limited by both a permit from the city of Toronto and Hong Luck's physical resources. With enough participants to sustain them, I have seen Hong Luck parades go as long as six-and-half hours, which included patrons not only on the main streets, but also in Chinatown's two main shopping malls: Dragon City [*Lùhng Sìhng*, 龍城] and Chinatown Centre [*Màhn Wàh Jūngsām*, 文華中心]. While in Hong Kong in 2012, I observed a Chinese New Year lion dance parade at the large IFC Mall for comparison. Although there were half as many businesses compared to the Spadina/Dundas area, participation levels from patrons was near one hundred percent, so the number of performances was around the same. This parade might have gone on for as long as one of Hong Luck's were it not for the smaller space and the deployment of two full lion dance teams working simultaneously. The result was that the IFC Mall parade lasted just over two hours. My consultants at Hong Luck told me that in the old days they also used to send out two full lion dance teams for parades (including surplus performers to allow people to switch positions and take rest breaks). During my fieldwork, however, there were not enough able-bodied members trained in lion dance and percussion to field more than one team.

On the day of the parade, Hong Luck members old and new gradually start gathering at the club several hours before noon. The first arrivals tend to have responsibilities such as preparing the offerings on the altar, organizing the lion dance equipment, and distributing the flags carried by non-performing members.[6] Other people, particularly those who no longer train

---

[6] The day before a parade, senior members would often be at Hong Luck late into the night cleaning the inside of the building, festooning the outside with flags, inspecting/repairing lion heads, and preparing the instruments. These duties were in addition to passing out flyers for the parade, as well as organizing supplies such as bottled water, firecrackers, a large order of dim-sum buns, and a whole roast pig to put in front of Guan Yu's altar.

regularly at the club, might show up early just to socialize with old friends. As the building begins to fill up, the diversity of Hong Luck's membership becomes apparent. The group has people from ages five to eighty-five, including members from a variety of different ethnicities. The elders were all Chinese Canadian from the Southern part of China, but the younger generations are more multicultural, which reflects Toronto's diversity. Hong Luck Upstairs is usually well represented, and quite a few Hong Luck Kung Fu Club "graduates" return just for the parade.[7] When it is nearly time to start, the training hall resounds with the chatter of between twenty-five and fifty people. Not everyone joins the parade, however, as many of the elders are too old to walk around in the cold for hours at time. Furthermore, the number of participants varies over the course of the day as some people leave early and other people show up late.

In order to get the parade started, there needs to be a critical mass of participants, who are then mobilized by a sonic catalyst in the form of martial sound: gong and drum percussion, kung fu shouting, and exploding firecrackers. When it is almost time to begin, the percussionists warm up the room by playing their instruments, which in Cantonese is called "opening drum" [hōi gú, 開鼓] or "rising drum" [héi gú, 起鼓]. The drum opening serves as a warning signal, letting the group know the parade will begin soon. These mini-performances do not include any lion dancing, however, but they still use the rhythm patterns of a lion dance as the basis for ornamentation and variation. As mentioned earlier, a bustling atmosphere is valued in Chinese culture. The noisy percussion heats up the room, aurally setting the mood for parade participants. Notably, people do not stop their conversations during the opening drum. Instead, they speak louder, thus further increasing the overall noise level in the room. After the drum opening, there would be a pause for last-minute preparations, which at Chinese New Year meant participants putting on their outdoor winter clothing. Then, everyone lines up in several rows as the head instructor (or a senior member) lights incense on the altar. The whole group simultaneously performs kung fu bows, first towards Guan Yu's altar, then towards photos of the kung fu ancestors on the wall. The bows are punctuated by vigorous shouts, uniting the whole group in martial sound and signalling full readiness. Then the

---

[7] In a kung fu club, the hierarchy uses a pseudo-kinship model based on seniority, rather than the coloured-belt system used by many Japanese and Korean martial arts. Students therefore do not really "graduate" because there are neither exams nor formal rankings, although a master can grant advanced disciples the right to start teaching and open their own schools.

percussionists start playing again as the parade begins in earnest with two lions bowing at the altar, doing a short dance, bowing to the kung fu ancestors on the wall, and exiting the building. Outside the club, someone would light a string of firecrackers, which the lion dancers would "fight" with, aggressively shaking the heads while kicking and leaping from stance to stance. The percussionists play extra loud to compete with the firecrackers, literally starting the parade with a bang. From the drum opening to shouting bows to pyrotechnic explosions, successive waves of martial sound create a crescendo of energy that unifies Hong Luck members as a troupe and fires them up for the day's activities.

Martial sound is more than an accompaniment or supplement; it drives and organizes the action. When I first joined Hong Luck, I was excited about getting to participate in parades, but, after having done a few of them, the novelty wore off. It was replaced with a feeling of dread in the days before a parade because I knew just how much energy was required to lion dance and play percussion all afternoon in the freezing cold. The day after a parade, I was guaranteed to be tired and sore. Nonetheless, the pre-parade ritual banished any hesitance and filled me with energy. I was not alone in this energized reaction. A senior Hong Luck member told me that the familiar drum rhythms made her blood boil and her hair stand on end, indicating the visceral, embodied response that practitioners have to martial sound. The power of ritual action exceeds conventional symbolism because, as Steven Friedson suggests in regard to Tumbuka healing ceremonies, "[i]nterpretation does not arise from or flow out of experience; lived experience is, at its very inception, an interpretation" (1996: 5). Hong Luck members embody a reflexive understanding of martial sound's motivational qualities, responding to it energetically rather than through discursive interpretation of its ritual or historical meanings. Their stance on martial sound in the preparations before a parade is an answer to the call of the drum, which erupts in group shouting and explodes with the firecrackers.

Martial Sound and Parade Lion Dancing

Martial sound is key in supporting group cohesion, organizing ritual action, and providing energy during a lion dance parade. The percussion remains continuous throughout the day but varies in intensity according to the circumstances. The default rhythm pattern is the moderately paced "walking beat" [*hàhnglouh gú*, 行路鼓], which is particularly appropriate as the group moves from patron to patron. Lion dancers remain under the head but conserve their energy while in transit by minimizing their movements. The lack of choreography during the walking phase allows whoever is drumming to have more rhythmic freedom, helping to keep things interesting for the group. The most basic walking rhythm resembles a repeating "lub-dub" heartbeat that drummers return to in between variations. While the group is moving down the street, rhythmic variations help prevent boredom, but drummers also restrain their tempo and loudness to help everyone conserve energy. For performances, they play faster and louder to boost the group's spirit, but they also use more standard rhythm patterns to make choreographic cues clearer. I discuss the issues surrounding variation in more depth later in this chapter.

Lion dance requires teamwork, not only from seasoned performers, but also from junior dancers and from non-performers. Senior Hong Luck members walk ahead of the group to look for red packets in doorways and interact with patrons; after a performance, other senior members collect the money, keeping track of who gave how much and writing thank-you notes. When the lions arrive at a patron, someone would use hand signals to tell the drummer to stop playing a walking beat and cue the ritual performance. Similarly, the instruments usually stay outside on the street even if the lion(s) go inside to perform a more extended routine, which requires Hong Luck members to position themselves for a relay chain of hand signals to show the drummer when to play the rhythm cues. Novice lion dancers often get their first performance opportunities during parades, which Noah referred to as "on-the-job training." These events provide experience dancing a simple routine, and they also offer chances to play the gong or cymbals while more senior members play the drum. Intermediate or advanced lion dancers would usually take over for anything beyond the basic parade routine, such as businesses or tong associations that want the lions to come inside and pay respects at an altar. Nonetheless, beginners are sometimes under the head when a more complex routine is suddenly requested, and so they get on-the-job training through verbal and physical directions from senior students and teachers. Members who are less active as performers (usually from age or inexperience) can still support the core lion dance team by pulling the wheeled drum cart and/or holding the lion's tail.[8] Non-performing members carry

---

[8] The long parades through Chinatown are too taxing on Hong Luck's human resources to have a dancer playing the tail throughout. For most parade performances, one person animates the head

banners emblazoned with martial slogans and names of kung fu styles in Chinese, as well as the national flags of Canada and the PRC.

Individual parade performances always began with three bows as a greeting to the patron and a show of respect. The "bowing-lion" [*baai sī*, 拜獅] rhythm is a continuous roll followed by a pause and/or muted drum hit, which is repeated thrice. Next, the dancer lifts the lion head into the air, shaking it with short, sharp motions that make the fur, eyes, and ears vibrate. The "head-up" [*héi sī*, 起獅] beat is a steady stream of fast, even notes interspersed at regular intervals with grace-note rolls and is in double-time compared to the walking beat. The lion dancer then crouches down in preparation for "three-rises" [*sāam sīng*, 三升].[9] Starting low, the dancer shoots the head explosively into the air as s/he pops into a standing position, then drops back down into a crouch. As the name suggests, this movement is repeated three times and is matched to a rhythm pattern based on a short motif that is also played thrice. The final part of three-rises is a rhythmic cadence, at the end of which the lion dancer briefly poses with the head in the air. The martial sound for head-up and three-rises is loud and fast to engage the ritual function of dispersing negative energy; like cresting waves, the sound and movement in this section rises up and crashes down out of the more sedate walking beat. Then comes the plucking-the-greens sequence. It is accompanied by continuous, un-metered drum rolls for eating and a repeated rhythmic motif for swallowing,[10] which is followed by another rhythmic cadence similar to three-rises. Finishing with three-bows, the parade continues with a return to the walking beat.

I have provided a transcription of the rhythms for the basic parade routine, though this should be taken as a non-exclusive set of variations, rather than a prescriptive score (Figure 3.2). It is closest to the way that I play the drum, which is based on the style of my two main teachers: David and Noah.

and a second person merely holds the tail in their hands, rather than performing as the body/tail of the lion.

[9] Even Anglophone lion dancers at Hong Luck refer to three-rises by its Cantonese name *sāam sīng* [三升], although I have heard other clubs refer to it in English as *the shoot* or *shooting*.

[10] The younger generation of Hong Luck lion dancers preferred to do four swallows, while some older members insisted it should be three. Repeating the pattern four times has the advantages of ensuring there is enough time to vigorously spit the greens and of being symmetrical. Four is an unlucky number in Chinese culture, however, because the word "four" [*sei*, 四] sounds like the verb "to die" [*sei*, 死]. Some Hong Luck drummers split the difference by playing the rhythm four times but varying the timbre by using a different type of drum-stroke on the first one, thereby breaking up the inauspicious numerology.

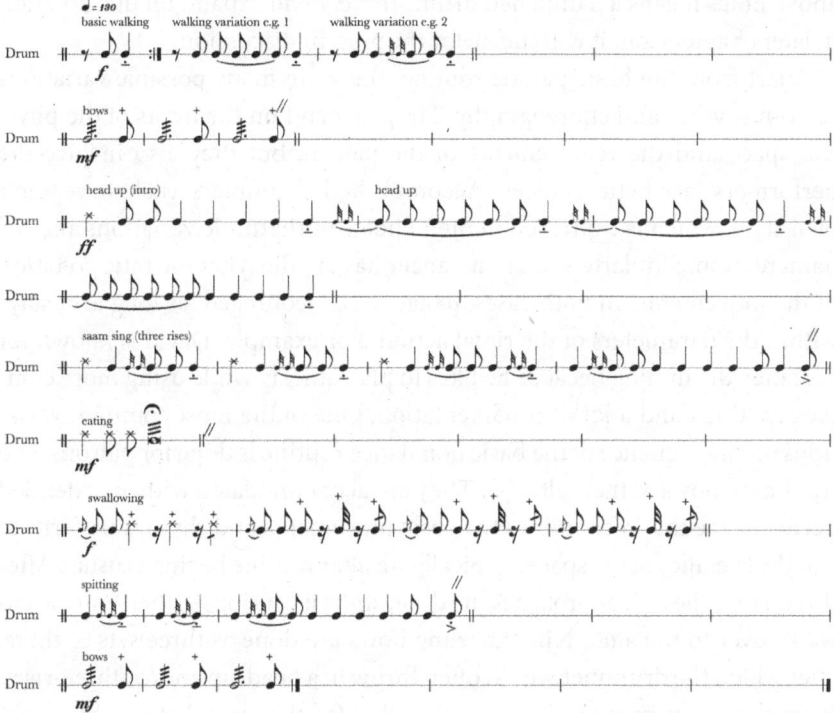

Figure 3.2 Transcription of Hong Luck's lion dance parade routine rhythms
Credits: Colin P. McGuire

Presenting it this way helps to avoid some of the issues with transcription that I outlined in Chapter 1. To summarize, my teachers were uncomfortable with the idea of anyone copying down rhythms from a recording, which David called "stealing learning" [*tāu hohk*, 偷學]. They preferred that I embody the beats by learning to play them and then write the transcription from memory. In fact, Noah forbade me from writing down the rhythms until I could perform to his satisfaction, including not only all the percussion parts, but also the lion dance. Reflecting the way these beats are experienced, I have not imposed Western time signatures, but have instead used duple subdivision, bar lines, phrase marks, and inflections to describe the drumming in a way that more accurately reflects an insider's understanding. The transcription contains only the main drum patterns and not the gong or cymbal accompaniment, but it does include indications for the lion movements associated with each section. The x note-head above the staff line is a rim click, the crosshatching on note stems indicates rolls, and the + sign above notes means a dampened drum stroke. I will expand on this notation in later chapters, but it will suffice for the present discussion.

Apart from the basic parade routine, there are many possible variations of both rhythm and choreography. These depend on the limits of the physical space and the requirements of the patron, but they also involve the performers' aesthetic choices. Accomplished drummers each have their own style, which is expressed in their choice of rhythmic variations and ornamentation. Similarly, each lion dancer has an idiosyncratic interpretation of the movements. In both cases, panache is encouraged, as long as it stays within the parameters of the ritual action. For example, David is known for his fancy drumming because he likes to play quickly while using more complex rhythms and a lot of ornamentation. One of the most common variations on the sequence of the basic lion dance routine is done for patrons who want nine bows at their altar(s). They are accommodated with an extended performance that recombines the basic movements and rhythm patterns to suit the specifics of the space. Typically, an altar routine begins as usual. After three-rises, the lion approaches the door, sniffs it cautiously, then enters, and walks over to the altar. Nine kneeling bows are done as three sets of three, after which the drummer would often throw in a head-up and/or three-rises. Patrons may or may not have a red packet for the altar that would trigger a plucking-the-greens sequence. After completing the altar ritual, the lion looks around for other altars (if found, the nine bows pattern is repeated) before backing out of the establishment to finish the routine by plucking the greens at the front door and giving a final three-bows.

As compared to the standard parade routine, there are two significant differences in the first and last lion dances of the day, both of which are done inside Hong Luck's training hall, facing Guan Yu's altar. The rhythms and movements are basically the same as the rest of the day's performances, but neither dance involves a plucking-the-greens sequence. Inside the club, lions pay respect to the tutelary deity without need for encouragement or payment. This situation indicates belonging, in the sense of being part of the group as well as being at home. The second distinguishing feature was the direction the lions face when entering and exiting a building. For parade performances, lion dancers enter face-first, but exit tail-first. On the one hand, this is respectful because—whether coming or going—the lion does not cross the threshold of the premises with its posterior towards to the patron. On the other, it is cautious as the lion does not turn its back on them, but rather keeps its vulnerable haunches towards the Hong Luck members waiting outside. When exiting Hong Luck to start the parade, lion dancers back out in a show of respect for Guan Yu. At the end of the parade the lions back into the club, which allows them to see who might be following them home into their den.

Ritual Protocols and Exceptions that Prove the Rules

Deviations from the established pattern of Hong Luck's New Year's parade stood out, underscoring the importance of ritual propriety through transgression. Such moments of disjuncture revealed the ongoing negotiation of lion dance as a living tradition. Hong Luck's senior members and patrons alike enforce protocols, so the specific context of Toronto's Chinese community has shaped the ritual over time. Some customs have gradually disappeared, while other aspects have proven indispensable. Complicated plucking-the-greens sequences that involve symbolic puzzles for lion dancers to solve were extremely rare during Hong Luck's New Year's parades, and some patrons dispensed with the greens altogether by simply hanging a red packet. A buddha character used to lead the lions during performances. This role was played by a masked person wearing monk's robes and wielding a fan; Hong Luck still has the mask displayed on a shelf, but it was not used in any performances during my fieldwork. I suggest that those parts of the tradition that are most actively maintained in the face of deviation present themselves as having special significance to audiences and/or practitioners. In this section, I look at issues surrounding lion dance parade conventions by considering several occasions when the usual patterns were disrupted.

Skipping or abbreviating parts of the pre-parade sequence generates uncomfortable feelings, which is not conducive to the lion dance's ritual function of dispelling negative energy. An example of truncated preparations occurred at the start of the Chinese New Year parade in 2011. Around 11:00 AM, the group had not yet finished organizing everything, when the president of the Hong Luck Association suddenly started rushing people out the door for a lion dance on the stage of the Chinatown Centre shopping mall at the southern end of the neighbourhood. While there was some resentment from performers that they had not been notified in advance, it was more of a problem because the opening sequence of actions at the club had been skipped. After the lion dance at the mall, which included a photo opportunity with local dignitaries, the group returned to the club to re-start the parade correctly. It was nearly 1:00 PM at that point, and the day was an hour behind schedule. It would have been more efficient to start the parade from the shopping centre, but senior members marched everyone back to the club in order to initiate the parade with an abbreviated version of the conventional opening. There was no time to open the drum or light firecrackers on the street, but incense was burned, kung fu bows were made (including martial shouts), and the lions did a rushed routine at the altar.

The state of the group remained scattered, which was manifested in the way the parade proceeded from this rocky start. Instead of the usual, orderly procession through Chinatown, we inefficiently forged ahead only to return a half-block to a store that had somehow been missed. Furthermore, the lion dancers' movements lacked their usual spirit, and the percussionists sounded erratic. Under the lion head, I struggled to follow the drum rhythms, which lacked the energy that they should have been imparting. I had to focus intently on the beats to hold onto the changing structure of each routine, rather than the rhythms driving me to move as they usually did. Everything felt laboured, and the usual pleasure I got from group performance was replaced with malaise. Several of my fellow performers commented on the chaos, attributing it to the lack of initiatory ritual. They revealed their stance on the importance of these protocols in their absence. The organizing and motivating effect of martial sound in the pre-parade sequence proved to be essential to not only a good start, but also to the overall trajectory of the day. It took over an hour before the troupe managed to pull itself together, although the energy was never quite as strong that day as it was during other parades.

Another example of disruption occurred during Chinese New Year 2013, when a large restaurant (i.e., the whole top floor of a building with a seating capacity over 500) requested an extended lion dance performance in the middle of the parade. Requests for special lion dances are not unusual; many patrons ask for extra actions beyond the basics, such as nine bows at an altar or for the lion(s) to walk around the interior of their premises. The problem was that the manager wanted far more: two altar routines (cash register and kitchen), a full-on stage show, and plucking the greens for any interested customer. The owner of the restaurant was affiliated with Hong Luck and the club usually held its anniversary banquet there, so the request was accommodated—despite the disruption to the parade. The lion dance team dutifully went upstairs, leaving non-performing members on the street. The customers obviously enjoyed it: a majority of them wanted a table-side plucking-the-greens with the veggies and red packets provided by the restaurant. The offer of a red packet required a minimum of three bows as gratitude and perhaps a bit of playful interaction, if not a miniature routine. The other lion dancer and I collected over thirty crimson envelopes of cash but spent nearly an hour inside the restaurant at a time when we should have been out on the street.

The interruption threw the day off for both Hong Luck and the other patrons in Chinatown. Non-performing Hong Luck members had to wait outside in the cold and, naturally, were nonplussed. Performers were dressed in layers appropriate for the wintry weather outside, so we removed as much clothing as we could before we started, but we were still massively overdressed for lion dancing inside. Consequently, we were drenched in sweat by the time we were done, which made our return to the parade outside very uncomfortable. Furthermore, the command performance was at a specific time that did not coincide with the parade route's timing and required a two-block detour with an eventual return to pick up where the procession had left off. Another large restaurant that normally got a lion dance for the New Year ended up rejecting Hong Luck even after we hauled all our equipment up the stairs to the second floor. The staff had heard the lion troupe pass by when we went to the command performance, and by the time we got to them, their lunch rush was already finished. They felt slighted by the favouritism shown to their competitors and snubbed Hong Luck out of spite. Finally, many other patrons got rushed performances because we had spent too much time inside the one restaurant.

Hong Luck's Chinese New Year parade has to be adjusted to make sure the space of Chinatown is covered within the limits of the club's human resources and the specifications of a police permit. When the parade protocol is distorted for one patron, it creates problems for both Hong Luck and other patrons. In the example of the special restaurant performance, the extra money was welcome but not worth the disharmony it created. The next year, Hong Luck coordinated with the manager to visit the restaurant in the morning before the parade officially started, thus removing the disruption to the procession while still satisfying social obligations. Similarly, Hong Luck had to turn down future invitations to perform at local malls on the same day as the parade, offering instead to do them on another day or referring them to affiliate lion dance groups.

Parade lion dance routines are stripped down to only the most essential parts in the interest of time, but there is a limit to how short they can be

before they start to lose their ritual efficacy and entertainment value. I sometimes observed over-shortening when there were not enough performers for
the rotation, when the day was almost over without having covered all of
Chinatown, and/or when the weather was particularly bad. Martial sound
organizes the ritual, so it was up to the person playing the drum to adjust
the choreography. Some drummers tried to abbreviate the already minimal
parade routine by leaving out three-rises and rushing through everything
else at breakneck speed. Patrons' negative reactions to over-shortening were
obvious from their frowns and the looks of disappointment on their faces,
as well as their anxious demeanours. The effect of a hasty lion dance was
rude (despite the bows before and after), because it was the equivalent of a
dinner guest who scarfs down their food and is already on their way out the
door as they are still chewing. In terms of ritual efficacy, the lack of three-
rises meant that not enough time was spent to fully disperse negative energy,
while the entertainment aspect also suffered from the reduction in rhythmic
and choreographic interest. A rushed plucking-the-greens often resulted in
the veggies not being well distributed when they were spit out. Ritually, the
greens symbolize wealth, so it is important for them to be in many pieces
that can be showered on the patron and/or their premises, not just tossed
out in a lump at the lion's feet. As the highlight of the performance, a vigorous plucking-the-greens sequence is entertaining because of the virtual
"explosion" of veggies, while a rushed one is anticlimactic. It is understand-
able that, when conditions were not optimal, drummers sometimes had to
rush parade routines (or were pressured to rush them by senior members).
Nonetheless, patrons were never happy with quick or lacklustre parade
routines—regardless of whether they took ritualistic or performative stances
on lion dancing.

   In order to improve efficiency during parades, Hong Luck's non-
performing seniors often encourage the lion dance team to do two patrons
at the same time. If possible, each of the two parade lions would do a ritual
for adjacent patrons simultaneously. It is a good way of speeding up the parade, but it can also cause problems when the routines are different, because
the gong and drum ensemble would have to play rhythms that only suited
one lion. The issue lies with the specific drum patterns that are used for each
section and the lion dance movements that go with them. For example, if
one routine occurred entirely on the street and the other required paying
respects at an altar inside, the rituals would diverge after the initial three-
bows, head-up, and three-rises. Advanced lion dancers could continue the

ritual without following the drum, but, in my experience, it feels terrible and results in a poor performance. Whereas martial sound both organizes movement and provides motivation, it can make things doubly difficult when one has to go against it by ignoring cues meant for the other lion. It is much worse for junior lion dancers because they rely more heavily on the drummer to guide their movement. In either case, the resulting performance is unlikely to satisfy patrons.

I have been involved with such problematic double lion dance routines in two capacities: initially as a performer and later as a team leader. During my first Chinese New Year parade in 2009, I was under the lion head and got confused when the drummer played a rhythm for the other lion that cued sniffing the door before entering a store. While that was happening, I was supposed to be plucking the greens, but I dutifully tried to follow the drum cue and enter my patron's store. Instead, a senior Hong Luck member shooed me back out to eat the lettuce, which I did while the drummer played a walking beat for the other dancer. Once I had the greens, I stopped dancing and waited for the other lion to pluck theirs so we could swallow and spit at the same time, but it took so long that I lost my concentration and missed the cue. It was probably the worst lion dance I have ever done. Fast forward to 2016 when I was a more advanced performer and also one of the team leaders. Twice during that parade, I stopped the group from doing simultaneous lion dance rituals because I ascertained that they would not be the same routine. I was nervous to contradict the senior members who were pushing for double lion dances, but they seemed satisfied with my explanation about how the ritual would be compromised by a lack of synchronization between lion and drum. Notably, Hong Luck members who have more lion dance experience do not call for a double ritual unless they know it would work, so I cannot blame the less experienced seniors who wanted to improve efficiency but perhaps did not understand the risk.

The first and last sequence in every individual parade routine calls for three-bows, which has proven to be both an immutable feature of the choreography and a fundamental part of the ritual. During a bow, the gong and drum ensemble plays a roll continuously in heterophonic unison. These bursts of rapid, evenly spaced sounds make a noisy-yet-organized texture lasting approximately one to two seconds per bow. The first roll is often preceded by a pause or a click of the drummer's stick on the rim of the drum as a cue, which the lion dancer(s) must respond to quickly. When these bows were not correct, patrons went as far as demanding that the ritual be restarted with a different lion dancer. During the Chinese New Year of 2009, for example, a relatively inexperienced performer responded late to the drum cue for bowing and made a flustered mess of the moves. The abbreviated first bow was followed by a second bow that caught the lion head on the store's awning and a cautious third bow that was totally unsynchronized with the percussion. The shopkeeper patron was much vexed after the dancer butchered these actions, and he pushed the lion back while shouting angrily. At that point, another lion dancer took over and the drummer recommenced the routine to assuage the concerned patron with a correct performance. It is rare for anyone to fully reject a lion dance, which points to the importance of the bows in establishing the correct frame for the rest of the actions.

Bowing is not an everyday part of contemporary Chinese culture (in Greater China or in diaspora) and is now primarily reserved for formal, ceremonial, ritual, and performance contexts. Lowering one's head embodies a stance on respect by assuming a subordinate physical position. In an extreme example, the "kowtow" [kautàuh, 叩頭] of Imperial China involved kneeling down and touching one's forehead to the ground in a posture of complete subservience. In modern times, bows are usually performed standing, with a motion that slightly lowers the upper body using a bend at the waist. I have observed and participated in a number of Chinese bowing practices both in Canada and overseas, some of which I will briefly describe in order to contextualize the types of activities that lion dance bows are linked to. In Hong Kong I had the opportunity to "pay respects on the mountain" [baaisāan, 拜山], which is a reference to the fact that Chinese burial sites are traditionally built on high ground. The most important time for this ritual is the Pure Brightness Festival [Chìng Mìhng Jit, 請明節], also known as Festival of the Tombs or Tomb-Sweeping Festival, which occurs fifteen days before the spring equinox. Relatives visit the final resting places of their forbears to bow, burn incense, deposit offerings, and/or clean the graves. Some Chinese people also bow when burning incense at altars to either ancestors or gods in their homes and businesses, as well as in temples. At Hong Luck, I became familiar with bowing at Guan Yu's altar when my seniors lit incense before class, eventually getting to light it myself when I began teaching.

Chinese martial arts involve a lot of bowing, far more than occurs in everyday life, which constructs and manifests a stance on them as a heightened type of activity. Hong Luck's kung fu bows were more elaborate than a simple bending at the waist, incorporating movement patterns from martial arts to form short pieces of bowing choreography. Various types of kung fu bows were performed before and after formal classes, as well as during the practice and performance of choreographed fighting skills. There is also a generic kung fu bow, common to many styles, where the clenched right fist is pressed against the open palm of the left hand with or without bending the upper body slightly at the waist. It is sometimes used as a greeting or acknowledgment among martial artists, as well as before demonstrations or competitions. Hong Luck members sometimes refer to this gesture as a Shaolin bow. The civilian equivalent has the left hand wrapped more loosely around the right fist while being rocked forward and backward.

Lion dance bows are slightly exaggerated versions of how Chinese people make a contemporary bow but with added martial flourishes in the footwork. To start and end a standard parade routine, Hong Luck dancers remained standing while rolling the lion head back, up, and down in a semicircle ending somewhere around their knees, which was sometimes abbreviated to a shallower bow during long parades. The kung fu posture for a basic lion bow rests on the "cat stance" [diu máh, 吊馬], which has most of the weight resting on the back foot and the front leg "hanging" or "empty" with just the ball of the foot touching the ground. The basic parade routine has six total bows grouped into two sections (three-bows at the start and three-bows at the end), but more bows were added for patrons that wanted the lion to come inside and perform nine-bows their altars. When Hong Luck's lions kowtowed at an altar, they used a "kneeling stance" [gwaih máh, 跪馬] with one knee down and the other leg bent. I have seen and done lion dances on parade that involved as many as thirty-three bows: three-bows at the start, nine-bows at the front door altar, nine-bows to an altar at the back of the business or in the kitchen, a further nine-bows at the cash register (with or without an altar), and a final three-bows after plucking the greens. The sheer volume of bows in such performances speaks to their importance. The significance of these actions connects with the type of situations in which bowing still occurs in Chinese culture, thus embodying a stance on bowing that gives the meaning of respect, propriety, and tradition.

Performing Identity through Lion Dance and Percussion

In this section, I discuss lion dance performance in the construction and expression of identity for Hong Luck, its members, and their patrons. The lion dance is certainly entertaining, but it is more than just entertainment.

Martial, athletic, choreographic, and theatrical aspects are all part of the ritual, helping to account for the widespread appeal of this practice beyond ceremonial exorcism contexts. When people take stances on lion dance that focus on affinity, culture, and heritage, they do not negate its function as a ritual, but rather build other values onto the para-liturgical foundation. In cases where people are less concerned about ritual propriety—or even ignorant of it—the performance's role as a marker of identity can even supersede its supernatural function. During my fieldwork, performing identity was as important for Hong Luck members as it was for patrons, but in different ways. When a performance offers several different meanings simultaneously, the result is semiotic richness, not contradiction, because the meanings are not mutually exclusive.

Lions are literally the public face of a kung fu club, and practitioners take a proud, protective stance on their masked costumes as the embodiment of their fighting spirit. I do not think it is coincidental that lion heads embody martial group identity and that one's honour or reputation in Chinese is called "face" [*mihnjí*, 面子]. In order to give, receive, and preserve face, there are protocols that must be followed when the lions from different Chinese martial arts groups meet. Senior Hong Luck members told stories about brawls over lion dancing between rival kung fu clubs in Hong Kong during the mid-twentieth century. Those recurring problems apparently caused public performances to be banned for several years. In Toronto, City Hall issues parade permits and typically—but not always—schedules kung fu clubs to do their parades on different days, perhaps to avoid problems like they had in Hong Kong. The Hong Luck Kung Fu Club was neither the only lion dance team in Toronto, nor was it the only group to perform in the Spadina/Dundas Chinatown, and I observed several occasions when kung fu lions met on the streets.[11] Herein, I focus on one particular example.

The local branch of the Chinese Freemasons has its headquarters two blocks east of Hong Luck on Dundas Street West, and they provided my first experience with intersecting lion dance parades. Master Paul Chan was a member of the Chinese Freemasons, and relations between the two groups were cordial. Their association hosts a kung fu club that also lion dances through the neighbourhood for Chinese New Year. Typically, each group would make a respectful courtesy stop at the other's building during

[11] During my fieldwork, there were at least twelve active kung fu clubs offering paid lion dance services in the Greater Toronto Area. This number does not include school programs or community groups who performed on an amateur basis.

parades. Regardless of good relations between the organizations, the air fairly crackled with tightly controlled martial energy when Hong Luck and the Freemasons somehow ended up doing their parades on the same day during Chinese New Year 2009.

When the two groups met, members on both sides visibly adjusted their stances on lion dance from celebrating the New Year to representing the martial ethos of their respective kung fu clubs. Hong Luck and the Chinese Freemasons were heading in opposite directions on the same side of the street, meaning their paths had to cross on the narrow sidewalk. As we approached each other, I could read dynamic tension in the trained martial bodies on both sides: hands raised, eyes narrowed, and postures grounded as people adjusted their physical stances to take a stance on readiness for action.[12] In that moment, my heart began pounding as I realized we were one false move away from a fight. The scene also revealed latent meanings for the non-performing members on parade. Seniors in both groups carried wooden staffs that they used as impromptu pedestrian barriers to make room for lion dancing on the narrow sidewalks, but these reverted to being martial polearms in the presence of another kung fu group. The throngs of martial artists carrying flags and banners were no longer ceremonial colour guards for their respective kung fu clubs; they reorganized their stances to emphasize being a show of force backing up the lions. In actuality, a martial stance on lion dance always undergirded these parades, but it was usually secondary to auspicious ritual action and festive celebration. The encounter did not change people's stances on lion dance as much as it revealed how the ritual is always-already a form of martial display.

Thankfully, there were no problems that day because Hong Luck and the Chinese Freemasons showed each other all due respect as their parades crossed. The dancers from both clubs kept the lion heads low and refrained from making sudden or aggressive movements, while the drummers led their respective gong and drum ensembles to slow tempos, basic rhythms, and quiet volume. The combined effect of movement and sound was one of deference, whereas raising the lion heads into the air with powerful drumming would have been a sign of dominance and thus a challenge to fight.

In contrast, I saw a lion dance at the Chinese University of Hong Kong in 2012 that purposefully used aggressive lion dancing and martial sound

---

[12] In theory, everyone in a kung fu club can fight, though in practice people vary in experience, ability, and interest with regard to the practicalities of hand combat.

as part of an intra-collegiate rivalry. There was a tradition within Chung Chi College of a lion dance group from one of the student residences going around to the other constituent residences of the college to exchange good-natured insults and taunts. In the winter of 2012, they visited the student residence where I was staying. It was after dark when they approached. They had a mass of supporters and began their visit with an "assault" featuring a black-and-green Zhang Fei fighting lion dance accompanied by heavy gong and drum percussion beats. The performance was followed by one of the marauders launching a volley of prepared invective, which was answered by a representative from the residence where I lived. Both groups had raucous support from their own members and suffered loud jeering from the opposition. It was all very collegial, stoking the fire of intramural sports rivalries and eliciting a great buzz from participants.

Practitioners of Chinese martial arts would have taken a very different stance on the event I observed in Hong Kong. Judging by the standard of their performance, none of the students practised kung fu,[13] and so they deployed martial posturing from a playful stance. When I returned to Toronto, I asked Noah what would happen if another kung fu club came to Hong Luck and acted as the student lion dance group had. He replied, "there would be blood on the streets," emphasizing that a Zhang Fei fighting lion and aggressive martial sound would have been bad enough, but the taunting would make a response mandatory. When the Chinese Freemasons visited Hong Luck at New Year's, they would first perform a typical parade routine outside. While the form and structure of their New Year's lion dance may have resembled what the students in Hong Kong did, the intention was different. The Chinese Freemasons were dispersing negative energy to make way for good fortune. The student group was building tension and rivalry, effectively sowing pugnacious energy without any real threat of violence. Furthermore, the Chinese Freemasons did the opposite of hurling insults after their lion dance. When they entered Hong Luck, their lion dancers literally crawled on their knees across the training floor to bow at Guan Yu's altar. The percussion that accompanied these extremely respectful performances inside the club was soft and subdued, using restraint of martial sound to show they were honourable by giving Hong Luck face.

---

[13] I later enquired where the student performers learned lion dance and found out that a kung fu master had taught it to their residence years ago. Ever since, each successive generation of students had passed on the lion dance to the incoming cohort.

If lions are the face of a kung fu club, then drumming is the heartbeat. Martial sound makes the collective identity of a kung fu group audile in much the same way lion dance embodies it, but drummers are accorded slightly more leeway in stamping the tradition with their own personal interpretations. Other types of traditional Chinese music also privilege the variation of shared repertoires, which is related to constructing the self-image of individuals, ensembles, and lineages relative to the broader streams of tradition and practice (Witzleben 1987). I heard repeatedly from Hong Luck members that no two drummers play the same way, and I learned to tell who was playing the drum without being able to see them during parades. I mostly based my recognition on their preferences for certain types of rhythmic variations and their use of ornaments. One senior Hong Luck member even claimed to be able to know who was drumming upon hearing the very first drum-stroke. The parameters most commonly affected by personal interpretation include rhythm, dynamics, accentuation, timbre, ornamentation, and embellishment, but more advanced players also create new rhythmic variations and manipulate phrase length for creative effect.

Hong Luck's drummers improvise frequently, according to both their technical ability and the performance conditions. When I write *improvise*, I mean it in the sense that Bruce Benson uses it (2003), referring to an "improvement" of the musical materials in real time through performance. Heard from this perspective, all musicking is improvisation and therefore does not need to be unfettered extemporization to qualify, which deserves some consideration in general terms. Along the same line of thought, notable jazz saxophonist Lee Konitz has identified a continuum of improvisation with ten levels that starts from playing the standard version of a piece, goes through increasing amounts of embellishment, and eventually arrives at "an act of pure inspiration" (cited in Kastin 1985: 56).

When accompanying lion dance performances, Hong Luck drummers need to stay on the first half of Konitz's continuum in order to make sure the sonic cues are clear and the rhythms match the choreography. Drummers typically avoid playing the most basic, unembellished beats because it would be boring for both performers and audiences. Nonetheless, they are circumspect in their improvisation when accompanying lion dance, restricting themselves to selecting from among a shared pool of stock rhythmic variations and adding their own ornaments or minor embellishments.

When the members of the gong and drum ensemble play without accompanying lion dance or kung fu (e.g., in the warmup before parades), drummers have more freedom, of which some of them take advantage by stretching their creativity. Unrestricted by choreography, they can play with the expectations of informed audiences by varying the sequence of rhythms to improvise structure, extending or compressing rhythms to manipulate phrase lengths, and using a greater quantity of variation. That being said, not all drummers can improvise freely. During my fieldwork at Hong Luck, David was most notable for being able to play on the freer side of the improvisation continuum that Konitz has identified.[14] He sometimes reached to the sixth or seventh gradient, where his embellishments changed the rhythms to become something new while still referencing the standard pattern. For example, if he played a fancy walking beat, it was still recognizable as a walking beat, but he could generate new variations of it on the spot. He also knew a wider range of rhythmic variations than most drummers, allowing him to string together longer combinations of stock patterns without repetition.

The combination of rhythms chosen and way of embellishing them are the hallmarks that characterize a drummer's personal flair, which must still remain within the framework of group sonic identity. Drummers have to know and respect the bounds of Hong Luck's tradition, as well as the broader Futsan versions of Cantonese lion dance drumming. Martial sound can thus be heard to perform sonic identity in a series of circles that expand from the individual, to the group, to the style. When these circles align, they share a common centre that makes them concentric. This alignment connects drummers and their audiences to sonic patterns that are identifiable, thereby constructing identity through martial sound structures of sameness modified by acceptable creative difference.

Martial sound can be used to include or exclude people, and so there are practical reasons for drummers to rein in their personal creativity and attune their playing to the community of practice. Inclusion and exclusion have to do with both ability and knowledge. For example, Master Jim praised David's drumming but also occasionally scolded him for playing too fast, too fancy, and too free. When the cymbalists, gong player, or the lion dancer(s) cannot follow the drum rhythms and/or keep up with the tempo, a drummer is excluding them with virtuosity. On the other hand, when a drummer works with a skilled, experienced lion dance team, virtuosic playing creates an elevated moment of performance in which not everyone could participate.

---

[14] In the past, an elder named Frank Ng was also noted for drumming skill and ability to improvise. Unfortunately, he was no longer regularly active by the time I joined the club.

During parades, inclusion relies on sticking fairly close to Hong Luck's shared tradition in terms of using the most well-known rhythms. These events bring together members from different generations who do not regularly perform together. In such situations, there is less tolerance for individual flair because it could be difficult for people to follow. When inclusive playing is required, judicious embellishment is more effective than freer forms of improvisation. Parades foreground group identity over personal expression.

Adherence to group tradition marks insiders and outsiders, making martial sound a way of showing belonging—or lack thereof. For example, during the Chinese New Year parade of 2014, a person whom I did not recognize tried to join the lion dance parade but soon revealed that he was not a Hong Luck member through the way he played the instruments. It was not unusual for an old member to come to the parade after a long hiatus or for senior members with their own clubs to send their students to help, which is what I assumed was happening. Hong Luck's non-performing seniors are normally good at preventing lion dance audiences and random pedestrians from interfering with the parade, but the interloper insinuated himself gradually enough to escape their notice. He followed us for several blocks, moving closer and closer to the instruments. When one of the cymbal players got tired and looked around for a replacement, this fellow was right there to take over and could play the supporting patterns in an acceptable fashion. Afterwards, senior members told me they realized the interloper was not Hong Luck when he started playing, but they let him continue because he fit in well enough that he might have been a student from an associated group.[15] When the interloper managed to get on the drum, however, it became apparent that he was an outsider. Although he could play Futsan beats, he did not know Hong Luck's characteristic rhythm patterns or the club's lion dance parade routine. Even patrons noticed the disjuncture, turning towards the interloper with scowls on their faces. A senior member ordered me to take over and not to let him play anymore, which I did post-haste.

On China Day in 2010, I witnessed another example of martial sound being used to represent Hong Luck's identity through marking insiders and outsiders. The club was participating in a flag-raising at Queen's Park (provincial parliament building) for the PRC's national day. About an hour before the ceremony, a group of elders proudly wearing their Hong Luck jackets

---

[15] There was a rumour that this person had learned from the Chinese Freemasons, but I was not able to confirm this.

met the lion dance team near where the flag would be raised. Although they were not performing that day, the elders wanted to open the drum, which was a rare opportunity to hear them play. A group of them, including Master Jim Chan, took turns on the gong and drum instruments, rotating roles but keeping the beat continuous. They played some variations that I had not heard before and put a different spin on familiar rhythms, showing the roots of Hong Luck's style. Eventually one of the elders bellowed "young men!" and Hong Luck's current lion dance team began swapping in on the instruments, which revealed both acceptable stylistic variation and how rhythmic identity is policed. The energy of youth was expressed in noticeably greater loudness and speed. The sonic texture was also more clearly defined but less full because of the way Hong Luck's younger members used articulation. While the elders tended to allow the percussion instruments to ring, the younger performers tended towards a more staccato style, especially on the drum and gong. David showed off some of his fancy beats, eliciting nods of approval from the elders, who then began joining back into the rotation on the instruments. Then someone played an international-style Hoksan beat on the drum. This drummer was there to help out with the lion dance, but he was a student from a different club that was run by a senior Hong Luck member. The non-Futsan rhythms drew a pointed reaction from one of the elders, who stopped playing and put his cymbals on the ground, rather than passing them to another person. As he turned his back on the drummer, he made his stance on those rhythms clear: they were not Hong Luck. I asked Noah and David about it afterwards, and they both said they had seen similar policing of sonic boundaries through negative reactions to—or active discouragement of—rhythms that fell outside the club's tradition.

The lion dance is a marker of identity for patrons, too. I have observed that weddings remain an important occasion for the lion dance, but some Canadian-born Chinese or people of mixed Chinese ancestry are not particularly fussed about the ritual aspects. These patrons equate the lion with Chinese-ness and wish to express that identity at their nuptials through entertainment for their guests. The fact that such people still feel it is important to have a lion dance because of their heritage—even when they are relatively unfamiliar with it and sometimes mistakenly call the lion a *dragon*—speaks to the enduring power of the performance's role in constructing identity. In most cases, clients who lack an understanding of lion dance protocol defer to Hong Luck's experts on matters of propriety. Sometimes, however, patrons request changes to the performance that are meant to express their individual identities through the Chinese lion dance, but which conflict with the tradition.

For example, a bride and groom who wanted Hong Luck to perform at their wedding reception in 2010 requested that we use a progressive rock song instead of the gong and drum. The couple had a deep personal attachment to the song and little experience with lion dance, so they saw no problem with mixing ritual and rock. The groom was one-eighth Chinese and wanted a lion dance to honour that part of his heritage. To him, it would be entertainment and a performance of identity, but he felt that the sonic aspect was fungible. His stance on the lion dance took it as a token from a culture that he was only loosely connected to and largely unfamiliar with, so it was not surprising that he focused on the costume and movement as the more obvious symbol. The request was made months in advance, which allowed time for debate among the lion team. The consensus was that lion dancing to progressive rock was wrong for two main reasons: first, it was not Hong Luck's beats, and second, it was not an appropriate substitution. The additive meter in the tune conflicted with the characteristic movements of the dance and would leave the lions without guidance from the drummer. Furthermore, weddings are happy events requiring an auspicious performance, but my teachers deemed the timbre of the distorted guitar and aggressive singing to be too dark and angry-sounding for a lion dance. In the end, a solution was negotiated with the bride and groom. The lions entered the room and mingled with the crowd while the rock song was playing, but then we proceeded to do a traditional performance with our own gong and drum. This compromise satisfied the couple's desire to represent the groom's Chinese-ness alongside their identity as rock music fans, but it also allowed Hong Luck to maintain the standards of ritual propriety and the character of their lion dance. Such fraught negotiation is a somewhat extreme example, but it illustrates nicely how diverse stances on the same performance can construct non–mutually exclusive meanings.

Lion Dancing and Martial Sound in the Construction of Chinatown

Lion dance plays an important role in transforming the physical space of the Spadina/Dundas area into Chinatown as a social space in multicultural Toronto. The work of claiming places and making spaces is a common diasporic experience, and musical sound often plays a crucial role (Wrazen 2007). Before Chinatown moved west from its original location in the 1960s (as described in Chapter 2), the neighbourhood where it now sits had a largely Jewish population. The architectural style of the area is similar to adjacent districts of Toronto and was well established before it became Chinatown, although there are now two buildings that feature Chinese characteristics such as overhanging tiled roofs with upturned corners and pairs of stone lion statues guarding the doors. The Hong Luck Kung Fu Club's regular lion dance parades help to enact Chinatown's identity by performing culture in the streets. Similarly, anthropologist Anne Raulin has written about Paris' Little Asia that, "in a foreign metropolis, a pluri-cultural one at that, the Lion Dance celebrates thusly a sense of territoriality" (1991: 47).

Martial sound is essential to the way that Hong Luck defines the space of Chinatown through lion dance parades; it loudly announces a Chinese Canadian presence. While not all residents of the area are patrons, no one could avoid the thunderous gong and drum ensemble. The sound pressure level created by this type of percussion can be as much as 105 dB, which is as loud as a jackhammer breaking concrete. Hong Luck's gong and drum ensemble draws on its ancient origins as military percussion to sonically patrol and reinforce the neighbourhood's boundaries during parades. The rhythms signal lion dance choreography, rather than troop movements, and the bellicose timbres cut through urban traffic noise, rather than the din of a battle. The sound of the percussion fills the streets and can even reach inside buildings. Given the deplorable history of Chinese exclusion in Canada, asserting presence through martial sound is an empowering act. Hong Luck uses gong and drum to state "this is Chinatown," announcing the steadfast being of Chinese people and their culture in the Canadian soundscape. This sonic identity is most obvious to Hong Luck members and their affiliates, although it might not be quite as clear to a random passer-by. Nonetheless, upon hearing and seeing lion dance in the context of Chinatown, many people would quickly make the connection to Chinese culture.

The distinctive Southern Chinese lion was also materially present in the neighbourhood throughout my fieldwork. There were decorations, knickknacks, and souvenirs in the local shops such as lion puppets, dolls, and statues, as well as child-sized lion-head costumes (e.g., Figure 3.3). There was even a lion graffiti sticker, as seen on the back of a stop sign in Figure 3.4. Most significantly, lampposts along the Spadina/Dundas corridor bore flags

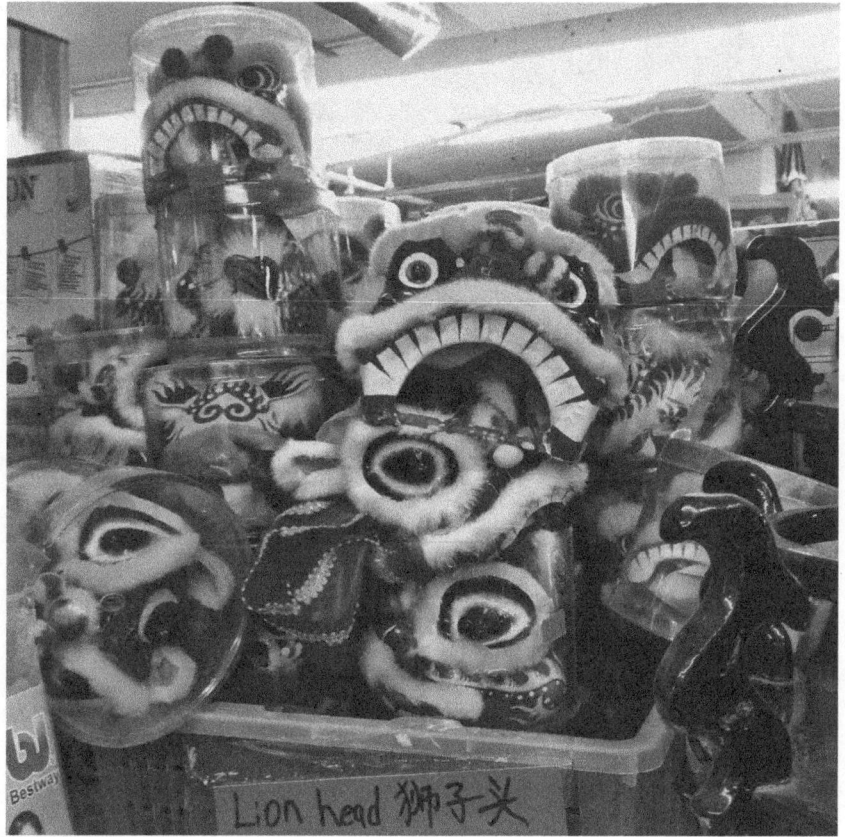

Figure 3.3 Mini lion heads for sale in a shop
Credits: Colin P. McGuire

with the image of a red and black Guan Yu lion and the words "Welcome to Chinatown" (see Figure 3.5).[16] A local group called the Chinatown Business Improvement Area [*Dōlèuhndō Wàhfauh Sēungyihp Chūkjeun Kēui*, 多倫多華埠商業促進區] sponsored these decorations, subsuming the neighbourhood's diversity of old and new Chinese migrants, as well as non-Chinese residents and businesses, under the image of a Cantonese lion.

Lion dance, martial sound, and kung fu in Chinatown have deeply social meanings, providing a role for people who might not otherwise be able to

[16] The lamppost banners defaulted to the "Welcome to Chinatown" lion, but also included Chinese lanterns made from LED lights and advertisements for Chinese cultural exhibits that held at the Royal Ontario Museum or the Art Gallery of Ontario.

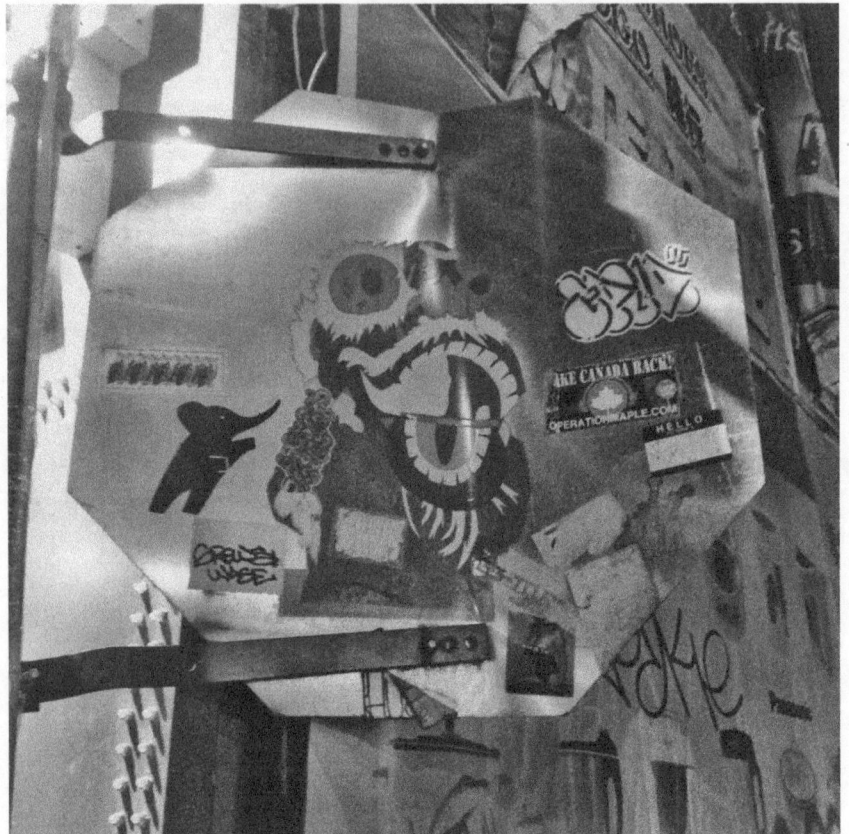

Figure 3.4 Lion graffiti on the back of a stop sign
Credits: Colin P. McGuire

integrate into the local diasporic culture and weaving them into the fabric of the community. The neighbourhood is no longer the Cantonese enclave it once was because migration from China has grown more diverse over time and there are also many non-Chinese people living/working there, too. Furthermore, Chinese people have spread throughout the Greater Toronto Area, delocalising the community. In the early twenty-first century, Chinatown is not merely a geographic place, but rather a space of relationships and culture that transcends its history as an ethnic ghetto. Writing of Toronto's Chinatown in the 1980s, Thompson suggested that

Chinatown may be viewed as a social system, separate from but linked to the larger Canadian system, consisting of a set of social positions and their

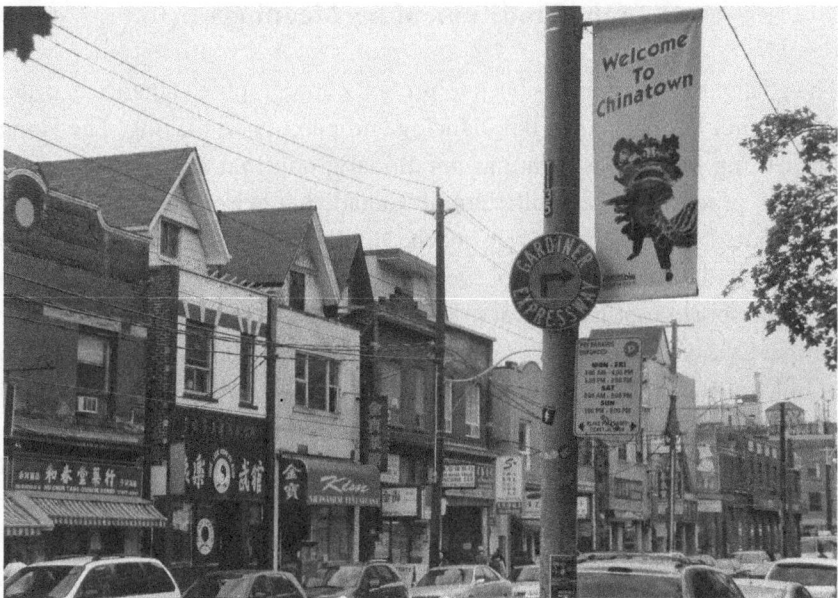

Figure 3.5 "Welcome to Chinatown" banner
Credits: Colin P. McGuire

corresponding roles. These statuses and roles are minimally defined by Chinese language and culture. That is, in order to participate in the Chinese community, one would have to possess the ability to fill an ethnic status (e.g., Chinese food cook) and perform the associated role (cook Chinese food in a manner acceptable to the Chinese owner and patrons). Since most Canadians do not have the linguistic or cultural ability to fill such positions, they are not members of the Chinese community. (1989: 26)

As a non-Chinese lion dancer, I had a path to become a participant in Chinatown society. Nevertheless, the ability to speak Chinese is significant, and my emerging Cantonese language skills opened up relationships that otherwise would not have been possible. I observed, however, that being able to fulfil a socio-cultural role in Chinatown did not necessarily require Chinese language skills. Some Chinese Canadian Hong Luck members only spoke English (beyond a few words or stock phrases in Cantonese) but regularly lion danced, played instruments, and/or demonstrated kung fu in the area. They were thus able to fulfil an important cultural role and make space for themselves as members of the community.

One Tradition, Many Meanings

The goal in this chapter has been to present ethnographic vignettes in order to interpret key aspects of lion dancing and percussion playing. The Hong Luck Kung Fu Club is a multigenerational group that has maintained its vibrant practices in a multicultural Canadian environment, which has contributed to a distinctive approach. Nonetheless, the group adheres to a larger tradition, and many of the issues I have raised will be common to other diasporic Southern Chinese kung fu groups, as well as those in Greater China. Ethnomusicologists are often concerned with both the preservation of folk musics and attention to continuity of change in these practices (Nettl 2005). In presenting Hong Luck's lion dance and percussion, I do not provide comprehensive transcriptions, descriptions, or recordings of movement and musicking. As I explained in the first chapter, my seniors at Hong Luck preferred to preserve their traditions orally and steered me towards description and interpretation over transcription and analysis. My discussion thus comes out of performance ethnography as a dancer and percussionist with the club, amounting to a lion's-eye view of their practices.

Hong Luck's distinct context lends itself to flexible interpretation because people take a variety of stances on ritual function, performance aesthetics, and meaningful identification. The club's elders, seniors, juniors, and associates, as well as patrons of varying backgrounds, engage in ongoing negotiation of lion dance in Chinatown and how it should be performed. People's stances on the practice determine their ideas about how it should be done and what that would mean. The contested signification process results in dialogue that can be contentious, but is not usually factious. In fact, lion dance and martial sound help to connect people across social, cultural, generational, and linguistic boundaries in Toronto. The exception to this general rule is the traditional exclusion of females demanded by some patrons, which has the potential to perpetuate sex-based discrimination and unequal constructions of gender. I return to this difficult situation in the next chapter, where I consider embodiment more deeply.

I suggest that the enduring value of lion dance has much to do with its ability to function on several different levels simultaneously, allowing people to take hybrid stances and adjust them depending on context. The traditional ritual serves as a para-liturgical blessing and exorcism, but it is also a performance of identity. For many patrons, a lion dance at Chinese New Year is essential for ensuring a happy, healthy, and prosperous future.

From a less mystical perspective, lion dance is used to represent Chineseness through banners, decorations, parades, performances, and sound that create the space of Chinatown and invoke cultural heritage at private events. For Hong Luck, the lion embodies the spirit of their kung fu club and brings together its diverse members to bond with one another through shared martial performance. Furthermore, the annual New Year's parade draws on kung fu meanings to empower performers and patrons, deploying a stance on Chinatown as a cultural space by claiming it from the Spadina/Dundas neighbourhood as a geographic place. Martial sound thus disperses the negative energy of historical Chinese exclusion in Canada through sonic strength, forbearance, and indominable spirit. The multiplicity of perspectives on lion dance in Toronto is not a problem to be resolved, but rather a source of its dynamism.

People's stances on lion dance and percussion are contingent upon a compelling performance, because a weak one lacks the energy required by the ritual, is unlikely to inspire feelings of identification, and is not particularly entertaining. A key source of lion dance's power is the training of its performers, which builds not only strength, endurance, and skill, but also embodied knowledge. The foregoing discussion of parades and performances has established a range of meanings, but these events are the tip of an iceberg compared to the bigger picture of practice. It is the week-in and week-out grind at Hong Luck where lion dancers and percussionists are forged. The next chapter heads inside the training hall, investigating the processes that transmit fundamental discourses about being a Chinese martial artist.

4

Kung Fu Apprenticeship and Embodiment

Introduction

In this chapter, I describe the experience of training at the Hong Luck Kung Fu Club in order to show how apprenticeship in Chinese martial arts and lion dance form the prerequisites to becoming a drummer. Overall, the transmission process has as much to do with becoming a well-rounded martial artist and community member as it does with teaching rhythms or instrumental technique. Relatively few people become drummers, because drumming is not taught per se, but rather emerges from transferable knowledge acquired through kung fu and lion dance. Briefly, students must do three things before they can be in a position to wield martial sound at the drum. First, they build a kung fu body, and second, they embody the lion dance. Third, they establish themselves in the community of practice, that is, a group of people with a common interest who improve their skills and knowledge through regular interaction with one another (Kenny 2016; Lave and Wenger 1991; Wenger 1998). Martial arts provide the physical foundation, and lion dancing inculcates rhythm, but to truly become a drummer requires being socially embedded in the kung fu club, because feedback from the community of practice is essential in shaping emergent drumming skills.

Bodily apprenticeship in kung fu, lion dance, and percussion is further complicated by two factors: gender and ethnicity. When Masters Paul and Jim learned martial arts in their Taishan county villages, the environment was very different from what Canadian students at Hong Luck experience in the early twenty-first century. In China, teachers and learners of kung fu alike used to be primarily male and Chinese. Now, more females and non-Chinese people have become involved, both at home and in the diaspora. Up until recently, however, tradition forbade females from participating in lion dance. I observed this gender taboo slowly changing at Hong Luck, including the first public performances of girls and women under the club's lion heads. Barriers to lion dance participation, however, slowed females' progress towards becoming drummers. The gender issue revealed limiting

Martial Sound. Colin P. McGuire, Oxford University Press. © Oxford University Press 2024.
DOI: 10.1093/oso/9780197775936.003.0004

assumptions about female ability and unmarked discourses about the masculinity of kung fu, all cloaked in the ritual propriety of lion dance. In a more inclusive vein, Hong Luck has accepted non-Chinese students since its earliest days. The club's mandate, however, is explicitly geared towards preserving and promoting Chinese culture, which has presented challenges for Canadian-born Chinese and non-Chinese Canadians alike. Embodying Chinese-ness through kung fu, lion dance, and/or percussion thus exceeds ethnicity, leading to hybrid, multicultural ways of being-in-the-world. I include discussions of gender and ethnicity in this chapter in order to show how becoming a Chinese martial artist intersects meaningfully with other aspects of practitioners' being.

Broadly speaking, this chapter is about doing as a way of becoming. I discuss what happens inside Hong Luck's training hall and reflect on my experiences of learning how to drum, which I compare with the experiences of my classmates and eventually my own students. First, I describe the inside of the club as a physical place to set the scene. Next, I analyze how (re)learning to stand and move in a kung fu way structures practitioners' being-in-the-world. Then I look at lion dance class and the ways in which it builds on the basics of kung fu, simultaneously teaching both movement and rhythm. The transmission process of kung fu and lion dance (re)constructs a Chinese martial arts body-mind—regardless of the practitioner's ethnicity. This new habitus opens the door to the drum, but crossing the threshold to become a drummer is up to the student. The final stage for prospective drummers is thus to gather embodied knowledge, translate it into martial sound, and actualize it on the drum. The whole community of practice then guides an emerging drummer's skills through both experiential learning and informal oral feedback, which I discuss relative to the network of social relations and pseudo-kinship structures of a kung fu club. I round out this chapter with considerations of gender in lion dance, attending to shifts in practice and performance in a multicultural, multigenerational, diasporic context.

The Martial Hall: Forge of Kung Fu

Hong Luck's "martial hall" [*móuhgún*, 武館] is narrow but deep,[1] with the main floor dedicated to teaching, learning, and training. As one comes in

---

[1] In general, Hong Luck's entire building is the martial "hall," but more specifically I am writing about the actual space where people practise kung fu.

through the south-facing, street-level door, there is a tight entryway created by a glass-topped counter on the left that cordons off a makeshift office. Under the counter is a mix of old and new uniforms, weapons, training equipment, gongs, cymbals, drumsticks, and "bruise liniment" [*ditdájáu*, 跌打酒], as well as copies of memorial booklets created for Hong Luck anniversaries. Just past the makeshift office space of the entryway is a small, carpeted area lined with chairs where people can watch the classes and/or socialize (see Figure 4.1). Photographs cover the walls of the entrance and sitting area: group shots from anniversaries; portraits of the founding masters; action shots of Hong Luck members; and souvenir photos of visits from celebrities and dignitaries, including former Canadian Prime Minister Pierre Trudeau, American kickboxing legend Benny "The Jet" Urquidez, and Hong Kong kung fu film star Jackie Chan.

Club members typically bow whenever they cross a thick, black line painted on the ground, which separates the linoleum of the training floor from the carpet of the social/commercial area at the entrance. They perform the bow facing towards Guan Yu's altar at the far end of the training hall, opposite the main entrance. The gesture signifies respect for the club and its

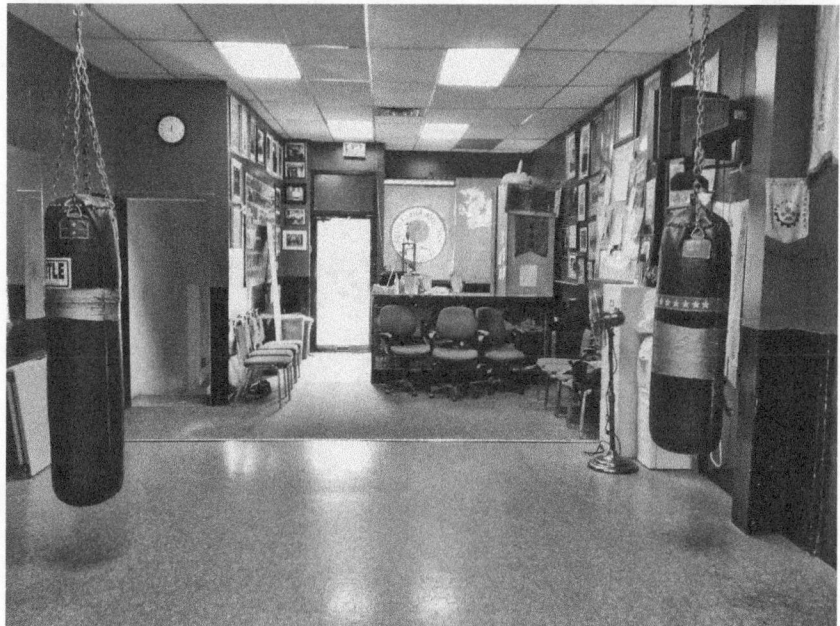

Figure 4.1 Hong Luck's main entrance and sitting area
Credits: Colin P. McGuire

kung fu, and it is the first lesson that new students learn when they join Hong Luck. Bowing at the line eventually becomes so ingrained that long-time members do it even when they are not there to train or teach, as for example when people come to visit or are collecting equipment for a lion dance gig. Whether as a slight movement of the head and/or hand(s) as they cross the threshold or a reverent pause marked by a deep bend at the waist with full Shaolin salute, the fundamental practice of bowing frames all activities on the training floor with a stance of respect.

The main part of the martial hall is an open floor that fills with moving bodies during training, but there is also a plethora of objects lining the edges of the space: training equipment, lion dance gear, memorabilia, and ritual implements. Just past the threshold of the black line on the floor, there hang heavy sandbags for practising full-power strikes (see Figure 4.2). The west wall to the left has two large windows and a door leading to the laneway outside, as well as two horizontal wooden bars used for balance while stretching

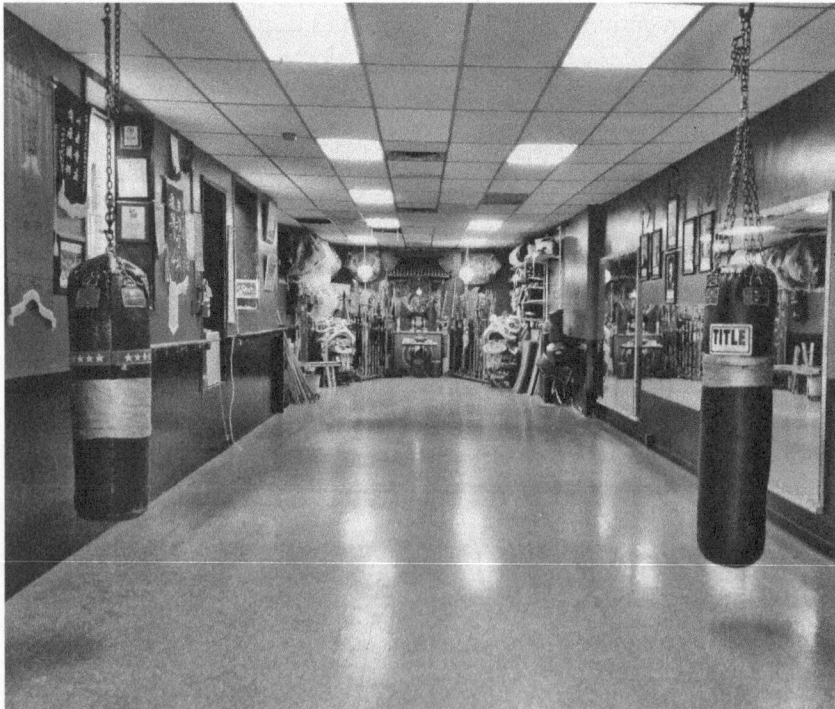

Figure 4.2 Hong Luck training hall
Credits: Colin P. McGuire

(like a ballet barre). Commemorative banners, plaques from tournaments, and photos of Hong Luck members festoon any available wall space. The right wall to the east has several mirrors that practitioners can use to check their positions during training, above which hang the portraits of departed masters from the club's lineage, including the founders of Choi Lee Fut and Do Pi. The back of the hall to the north is used for storage of various types of equipment, like grappling mats, free-weights, and striking pads, as well as the rolled-up flags and banners used for parades. At the end of the martial hall against the north wall sits Guan Yu's altar (as described in Chapter 3), which is flanked by two racks of Chinese weapons that extend at angles from the tutelary deity's dais. There are long armaments such as staffs, halberds, and spears; short ones like swords, knives, axes, and maces; miscellaneous implements used for martial purposes, including rakes, hoes, flails, and benches; and some truly idiosyncratic weapons like the paired, spiky, metal rings called "wind and fire wheels" [*fūng fó lèuhn*, 風火輪]. Behind the kung fu arsenal, older lion heads that are only used in class sit on top of beat-up practice drums, while the newer heads that are reserved for performances hang on the walls to either side of Guan Yu.

Hong Luck's building and furnishings, as well as the kung fu and lion dance equipment, are serviceable but a bit rundown, requiring ongoing maintenance efforts. The club is a registered not-for-profit organization, and volunteer labour is necessary for upkeep, as hiring a caretaker or contractors is not in the budget. Revenue from tuition fees goes only so far, especially given the rising popularity of mixed martial arts (MMA), which seems to have detracted from traditional kung fu's appeal among potential students. Furthermore, many senior members no longer pay fees at all, but instead volunteer as teachers, performers, administrators, and superintendents. Many members do basic cleaning and tidying, but some have also done full-on renovations like painting the walls, patching the roof, or refurbishing bathrooms. People also volunteer to work on Hong Luck's virtual presence online.[2] In addition to tuition fees, lion dance is the other main source of revenue.[3] Although performers sometimes receive an honorarium and usually get a meal after the gig, they volunteer their time and effort to help support

---

[2] http://www.hongluck.ca/.
[3] The club's income used to be supplemented by the activities of the Hong Luck Association, but this source of revenue has been smaller in recent years. The anniversary banquet and random donations from patrons also help keep the club going.

the club. Just as some members help with building maintenance, lion dancers end up repairing the heads and instruments.

Volunteer labour of all varieties is so central to Hong Luck's continued existence that it is part of what it means to be an active member of the community of practice. The collective effort is mostly self-organizing, rather than being the result of central authority or assigned duties. Anyone who has stuck around Hong Luck for a while has probably done chores. These contributions bind members to the club—and one another—through a sense of responsibility. The physical place and its materials embody the martial hall, such that membership incorporates a stance on duty to the collective body. For example, I have not only repaired weapons, fixed lion heads, built a gong stand, and taped drumsticks, but also shovelled snow, swept floors, dusted counters, taken out the trash, and replaced light bulbs. At first, seniors occasionally asked me to help them with whatever chore they were working on, obliquely helping me realize the necessity of volunteering. As I became more embedded in the club, I noticed tasks that needed doing and took responsibility for them. My contributions to maintenance, along with my performances as a lion dancer, were important to becoming a full-fledged member of Hong Luck. I gradually began to change pronouns, referring to the club in the first-person subjective plural (we), rather than second-person subjective plural (you). Around the same time, my consultants started to do the same, subtly actualizing my membership in the club through terms of address.

With a perpetual lack of funding, both the building and the lion dance equipment bear traces of members, past and present, inscribed through makeshift repairs, ad hoc overhauls, and repeated restorations. Hong Luck's slightly rundown appearance belies the amount of attention and care that members have put into it. After decades of cobbling the place together with donations, recycled materials, and volunteer labour, the whole building—from roof to foundation—has at some point had work done on it. While some senior members might remember who did what when, the collective stance on the martial hall tends to subsume individual effort into communal being. Hong Luck's community identity is even apparent in the place's aroma. For example, a new lion dancer once remarked on Hong Luck's distinctive odour: musty and dusty, spiked with a mix of incense smoke and stale sweat. Noah told her that it was the scent of the kung fu ancestors, whose presence pervaded the martial hall.

Forging a Kung Fu Body through Basic Training

During my fieldwork at Hong Luck, there were three beginner classes per week, which was where all new students began their training. In my first three months at the club, I tried to attend all three weekly beginner classes, although I then cut back to just one or two in favour of lion dancing and more advanced martial arts training. The instructors on Thursday evenings and Sunday afternoons varied, but Quang Thang consistently taught on Tuesday nights. I attended his class weekly throughout my first two years at Hong Luck. In this section, I describe Quang's class, which was relatively consistent from week to week and also very rigorous in terms of basic training.

Before all classes at Hong Luck, someone lights incense at the altar and does three bows towards Guan Yu; in the beginner classes this is the responsibility of the teacher. The other classes, including intermediate/advanced kung fu, lion dance, and sparring, are more relaxed about who lights incense because all the participants are already established members. Beginner classes, however, serve to induct new students into the community of practice and are thus more structured. Students usually arrive to Quang's class a little early to change into their uniforms (a Hong Luck T-shirt, black pants, and black waist-sash) and warm up before the two-and-half-hour workout. When it is time to start, Quang has students line up in rows and stand quietly while he lights incense and bows at the altar. Next, the whole class performs stylized Do Pi and Choi Lee Fut bows first towards Guan Yu at the back of the hall and then towards the portraits of the kung fu ancestors on the east wall. At the end of beginner class, everyone performs the same group bows but without the lighting of incense.

Beyond teaching the formalities of the martial hall, beginner classes also serve to restructure students' being-in-the-world through new ways of standing and moving. Basic training is thus more than physical; it calls for a body-mind shift. Quang invariably started our training sessions with the all-important "horse stance" [*sei pìhng máah*, 四平馬], and he also used it as the default position between practising other stances and techniques. Through repetition, this kung fu stance serves as a catalyst in the process of becoming a kung fu practitioner. While it may seem trite to reduce the basis of a habitus down to a single pose, it would be difficult to exaggerate the importance of the horse stance at Hong Luck (and many other types of Southern Chinese martial arts);[4] it is literally and figuratively the foundation of kung fu, lion dance, and drumming. I return to this point later, but, for now, suffice it say that re-learning how to stand is the point of entry to a new way of being.

Physically, the horse stance is a sort of squat with the feet planted about double shoulder-width apart. In choreographed forms and fighting applications, the horse stance can vary in depth and width according to the circumstances, but in basic training the horse stance is wide and deep. The ideal is for students to get their thighs parallel to the floor and to be able to hold the position for minutes at a time. Due to limitations of strength, flexibility, balance, and/or endurance, few people can achieve and hold the full archetypal horse stance. Nonetheless, holding any kind of horse stance quickly causes people's legs to ache, burn, and quiver. At first this type of training is a torment, but it builds self-discipline alongside physical ability. Gradually, students become more efficient and therefore more stable, finding their balance so they can sink powerfully into the position.

Hong Luck members often told me stories about the rigours of training at an unspecified point in the past (i.e., "back in the day") when new students did nothing but practise the horse stance for months on end. This restricted training regime was supposed to have tested would-be apprentices' dedication by seeing if they could endure simultaneous pain and boredom, while also building up their power and stamina. In Quang's intense beginner classes, we covered a full range of traditional basics: stances, footwork, strikes, blocks, stretching, and the sets of choreographed fighting movements known as "forms" [toulouh, 套路]. Less frequently, he also had us work with a partner to practise attack and defence or hit hand-held striking pads. Fortunately for me, it was only three months before my foundation was deemed acceptable, and Quang gave me permission to join the lion dance class. Such progress was quick by traditional standards, which was partly due to my previous twenty-five years of martial arts training, my level of physical fitness, and my dedication. My speedy promotion probably also had something to do with the fact that Hong Luck was short on lion dancers, and I had announced my interest in that regard.

The following passage describes a typical experience during my first two years at Hong Luck when I was regularly attending Quang's beginner class:

---

[4] Not all styles of kung fu focus as heavily on the horse stance, but variations of it are common throughout the Chinese martial arts world. Moreover, the horse stance is also found in other Asian martial arts.

Incense smoke begins to fill the air as we move through the Do Pi and Choi Lee Fut bows, then Quang calls for horse stance. We stand in silence, breathing through our noses with tongues pressed into the roofs of our mouths and focusing our eyes on the red light above Guan Yu's head. Quang barks "LOWER," then counts down ten seconds. Next, he calls for a forward stance. Again, we hold it, breathe, and go lower, before we return to horse stance. Barring the door stance. Horse stance. Sweat is starting to drip down my forehead and into my eyes, but we're supposed to remain still while holding stances, and so I try to ignore it. When Quang calls for the next pose, I quickly wipe my face as I transition to a sitting dragon stance. Horse stance. Girl stance. I try to push myself to go lower, to hold the position, to build my foundation. Horse stance. Kneeling stance. My legs are burning! Every fibre of my being is telling me to stop, but Quang is relentless. Single-blade stance. Horse stance. I'm living for the brief reprieves between postures . . . Cat stance. Horse stance. Always back to horse stance. Finally comes the crane stance where we get to stand up on one leg instead of having to sink down low! Horse stance. Sitting on a lotus stance. Horse Stance. Now Quang calls for footwork drills, requiring stepping and twisting from horse stance. And more horse stance.

Timing and synchronization are also important aspects of Hong Luck's beginner classes, and we did most of our training together as a group, organized by Quang's counting. After stances we worked on basic techniques, which we drilled in sets of ten, one count per move. At first, we moved in physical unison. The seemingly simple ability to coordinate our fighting skills as a group was complicated by our not always being able to see one another. Quang's verbal cues were therefore essential for keeping everyone moving in time together. Synchronization in this context means neither anticipating the count nor having a delayed reaction, but rather attuning one's movement to a pulse established by the teacher's voice as a form of martial sound. Quang often reminded us to follow his count mindfully, which he explained would improve our martial reaction time. For more complex combinations of fighting movements, the relationship between the beat of Quang's counting and our movement became more complicated. When practising two or more linked fighting moves, we would start each repeated sequence together, but proceed through it with our own personal variations of rhythm and tempo. The personal differences in timing were subtle because they had to fit within the basically steady tempo maintained by Quang's counting, creating a macro pulse woven together from many idiosyncratic micro rhythm patterns. In choreographed forms, longer combinations can be comprised of as many as five or six fighting movements; variations in rhythm and tempo became more pronounced when the sequences were more complex, but each section still started on Quang's count.

There are at least four reasons for synchronizing group kung fu practice. First, there is a question of safety when many people are practising together—particularly when those people are relatively inexperienced novices. Quang's beginner classes typically had between ten and twenty people, and it would have been dangerous for everyone to practise kung fu at the same time without rhythmic coordination. Second, it feels good to move together, creating energy from a sense of embodied camaraderie. As one of my beginner classmates remarked, our classes were at times exhilarating when everyone was punching, stepping, kicking, and turning together. When a new student joined the class, however, Quang had to do more explaining and correcting. These interruptions broke the flow of our teacher's martial sound, which my classmates observed made class more tedious. Being in time together during physical exertion promotes what historian William McNeil (1995) calls *muscular bonding*, which is a visceral feeling of interpersonal connection that people experience through collective rhythmic movement. McNeil notes that activities like dance and military drill are important ways of building and sustaining communities, enhancing a group's ability to cooperate. In Hong Luck's case, muscular bonding also helps to transcend barriers of language, age, and culture through the shared experience of synchronized action. The third reason for synchronizing kung fu training is that many aspects of hand combat rely on rhythm and timing. The ability to coordinate with another person's movements, as well as to maintain or impose asynchronous combative relationships, have important implications for fighting applications, which I discuss in the next chapter. Finally, performing movements in time with martial sound is a foundational skill for lion dancers. Hong Luck's beginner classes lay the foundation for being able to follow the percussion, building students' ability to synchronize movement to martial sound. As with many aspects of kung fu training, following a teacher's count is not as simple as it might seem.

Embodying Chinese-ness through Martial Arts

After about eight months of fieldwork at Hong Luck, I received my first lesson from Master Paul Chan, who at that point normally only taught advanced students. In my experience with Chinese pedagogy (martial arts and language), praise is hard to come by and criticism tends to be direct, frank, and honest—nigh unto blunt. Despite knowing how this style of teaching works, I was a bit surprised by the scolding Master Paul gave me that day. When I told my seniors about it, they explained that it was an honour to be chastised by the club's elderly co-founder because he no longer bothered with students unless he saw potential. Master Paul's lesson that day was about how Hong Luck's kung fu is meant to embody Chinese-ness by demonstrating a stance on culture through the generation of physical force. It was an important moment of transmission, although I did not realize the full implications until years later. I describe the experience below, which occurred during an open training session where I was working on a basic Do Pi form that had been giving me trouble in class:

There's only one other student on the floor, and I'm taking advantage of the rare free time and space to practise at my own pace. Suddenly, Master Paul walks into the club, which is a bit of a surprise. I carry on self-consciously as he takes a seat in the common area. After watching for a few minutes, Master Paul calls me over and tells me to sit down next to him. He appears thoroughly unimpressed and says, "your kung fu lousy." I'm crestfallen and weakly try to protest that I'm just a beginner, which he ignores as he continues his tongue-lashing. Master Paul tells me I'm strong-but-stiff and much too slow, but that the worst thing is that my movement doesn't look Chinese. Being a European Canadian, I expect his next comment to be about my ethnicity. He surprises me by saying that my kung fu looks Japanese!

Finished with his admonishment, Master Paul kindly offers me a few pointers. The elderly master is fired up, and I'm in rapt attention. It's hard to understand his mix of Taishanese, Cantonese, English, onomatopoeia, and gestures, but I'm determined not to miss a thing. Apparently, my strength is useless because it's slow. I need to be looser to go faster. But "issuing power" [*faat lihk*, 發力] isn't just about speed. He says that eyes, hands, and stance go together, and I'm getting the idea that "power" is more than physical. Master Paul says I need to strike with a more "vigorous spirit" [*jīngsàhn*, 精神]. He punctuates this point ferociously, giving a bloodcurdling yell and hacking a punch so fast I barely see it. Chills run down my spine as I sense my master's stance on martial power: fierce, committed, and dynamic.

To conclude, Master Paul tells me to "make it more Chinese" and sends me back to practising. He then turns his attention to the other student.

My classmate is Chinese Canadian but inexperienced with kung fu. I can't help overhearing Master Paul's words, as he tries to coach the novice's awkward attempts to do a form. "You're Chinese! You should know," says the slightly exasperated master. Clearly, my classmate doesn't know, but he struggles gamely until Master Paul gives up and tells him to just keep practising. It appears that Chinese-ness is more than skin deep when it comes to kung fu.

The lesson I received from Master Paul that day was explicit: I was to embody a Chinese way of being-in-the-world through kung fu. My task was partly a question of acculturation, requiring me to work towards becoming more of a cultural insider. A well-known Chinese martial artist, teacher, and author named Adam Hsu suggests that Western students could benefit from learning about Chinese culture through arts, philosophy, and language so that they can better "savor the unique flavor of China's martial arts and apply that knowledge to their practice" (1998: 116). His proposition is equally applicable to some members of the Chinese diaspora who grew up in Western(ized) environments. My task was also a question of receiving transmission, requiring sensitivity to the often-unarticulated qualities of what Tomie Hahn (2007) calls *sensational knowledge*. As Hahn argues in her ethnography of transmission in Japanese dance, the senses are paths connecting body and mind to cultural knowledge. Rather than putting intellectual theory into practice, this type of transmission between teacher and student cultivates practice that leads to embodied theory.

Three aspects of Chinese culture proved particularly helpful in savouring the flavour of kung fu and cultivating my practice. The first is locating the centre of the body in a point approximately two inches below the navel, which in traditional Chinese medicine and meditative practices is called the *dāantìhn* [literally: cinnabar field, 丹田]. Quang sometimes called for us to breathe into this point during horse stance training. While I knew about the daantihn before I started at Hong Luck, putting this theory into horse stance practice was easier said than done. Instead, sensational knowledge acquired through practice (re)formed my understanding of the daantihn concept in a way that just reading about it could not have. Gradually, I discovered that I needed to root myself by sinking not only my physical posture, but also my being. As David explained in lion dance class, the horse stance only becomes more comfortable when one can be truly balanced and stable in it. Practitioners orient themselves to the daantihn by shifting the body-mind down, occupying a lower centre of gravity in a way that makes staying in the horse stance feel normal. Doing so provides a grounded stance on being-in-the-world by quite literally bringing one's physical point of balance closer to the ground. David claimed that he could sometimes tell when people had strong horse stances, even when they were just walking down the street. Apparently, he could tell if they embodied a more stable, rooted, and solid way of being-in-the-world. If he can actually perceive these qualities, then long-term physical training appears to inscribe a way of being that is not only durable, but also transferable beyond the specific postures of martial arts.

The second explicit aspect of Chinese culture I had to learn to embody was the coextensive, equal opposites of "yin and yang" [*yām yèuhng*, 陰陽]. In Taoist philosophy, the interplay of these two powers undergirds all of existence such that they are inseparable, despite being in constantly shifting opposition. The dynamic power of yin and yang is symbolized in a diagram showing a half-black, half-white circle with each part swirling around the other and containing a dot of its obverse within it. It is telling that Hong Luck uses a yin yang symbol as part of the club's logo (see Figure 4.3). Many

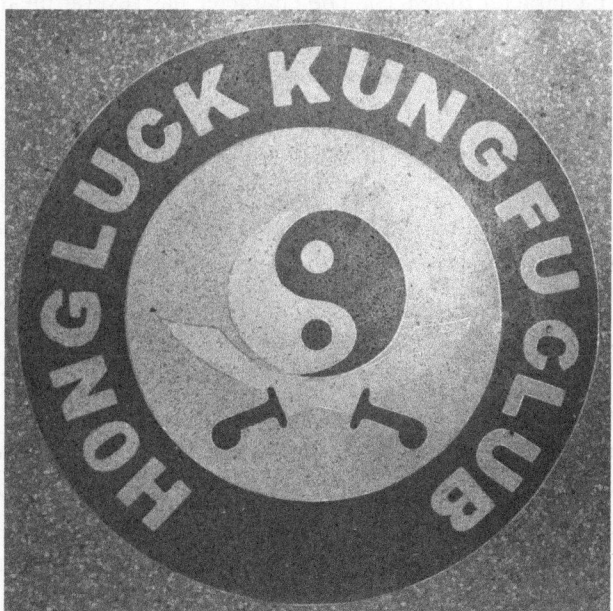

Figure 4.3 Hong Luck logo (set in stone)
Credits: Colin P. McGuire

kung fu techniques display a dynamic circularity, with actions balanced by their opposite as movements whirl around each other. Again, I thought I understood the theory of yin and yang from reading about it, but sensational knowledge taught me how the distinctions between opposites are mental constructs. Through kung fu, I learned what it feels like to simultaneously embody a balance of action and stillness, straight lines and rounded curves, speed and slowness, hardness and softness, and so on, which provided a lived experience of how yin and yang are co-extensive, not oppositional. Quang's beginner class drills these dynamics into his students through endless repetition, which helped me to realize the sensational knowledge required for martial arts performance.

The third way I came to embody Chinese culture through kung fu practice was with language and writing. At Hong Luck, teachers expect students to learn the Chinese names of techniques and choreographed forms, which people do with varying degrees of ability. Knowing the sound of the name is one thing, and understanding the meaning is another. To fully grasp the names of some postures, forms, and techniques, it helped me to know how to write them. For example, a forward stance with the front knee bent, the back leg straight, and the feet positioned at right angles to each other suggests the Chinese character *dīng* [丁]. The character has several meanings, but, in this context, it is its shape that matters; the stance is called *dīngjih máh* [literally: ding-character horse, 丁字馬] because the legs form a ding-like silhouette. Similarly, the "girl stance" [*néuih jih máh*, 女字馬] gets its name because the legs are crossed with knees bent into a shape that resembles the character for "woman/girl" [*néuih*, 女]. In some cases, it was the explanation of a technique that related to writing, rather than its name. A teacher who was visiting Hong Luck from China once explained to us that the angle of a certain swinging punch was like the top of the character *tīn* [literally: sky or heaven, 天].[5] Both the punch and the stroke used to write the top of the character have a slight downward curve that gently angles an otherwise horizontal motion.

The Chinese-ness that Master Paul was looking for in his students' movement also evoked writing through a gestural quality common to Chinese calligraphy, dance, and martial arts. The distinctive type of motion I am referring to involves a slight hesitation or slowing in mid-movement

---

[5] In some printed fonts, the top stroke of the character *tīn* [天] looks totally flat. In handwriting or traditional brush calligraphy, however, the slight downwards curve is more evident.

followed by a sudden acceleration that condenses force towards the end. This gesture is not just a phenomenon at Hong Luck, nor is it restricted to the Cantonese branch of Chinese culture. For example, dance scholar Lin Yatin (2010) has discussed the influence of both the gentle, slow, and flowing martial art of tai chi [*taaigihk kyùhn*, 太極拳] as well as Chinese calligraphy on Taiwan's Cloud Gate Dance Theatre. She notes that the spatio-temporal profile of martial arts and calligraphic brushwork ground choreography that "preserves and synthesizes a new Sino-cultural-based identity which draws on an ancient Chinese tradition and gives it a new location and embodiment" (2010: 259). In particular, she identifies how "the essence lies in the use of flow and its abrupt gathering of energy at the end" (ibid).

Before I was able to embody this Chinese gestural quality in Hong Luck's striking techniques, I learned to do it through calligraphy. While I was a student at the Chinese University of Hong Kong's Yale-China Chinese Language Centre, in 2011–2012, I observed how my calligraphy teacher's brushwork on each stroke of a character embodied a distinctive sequence of intentional movement: gentle-yet-firm initiation as brush touched paper, slowing to a smooth flow through the length of a stroke, and an accelerated condensation of force at the end to bring the brush out of contact with the writing surface.[6] These three phases fused together in the mark left on the paper, resulting in a record of intentionality: pressure, speed, and direction marked each part of a character but were most evident on the final stroke. While I cannot claim to be calligrapher, I was receptive to the timing and force my teacher accorded to his brushstrokes, which I came to recognize as being homologous with the way advanced kung fu practitioners strike. As with the last stroke of a character in calligraphy, the flowing/condensing quality is often exaggerated with a flourish on the final strike of a kung fu combination.

Learned habits are culturally significant to the habitus of members of a society, helping to explain how Master Paul perceived the flowing/condensing calligraphy-like movement of kung fu striking as Chinese. As per Bourdieu's (1990 [1980]) ideas about practical logic, the embodied dispositions of a habitus are transferable between practices, resulting in an economy of structuring structures. I may have had my first realization about this Chinese gestural quality through calligraphy, but I actualized it more completely in kung fu.

---

[6] In a short dot [﹨], the middle phase of the motion would be truncated, while in a more complex stroke [乙] the middle phase might include direction changes that would require a re-initiation without removing brush from paper.

Doing so helped me to modulate my striking with the flowing/condensing energy that was required to perform choreographed forms in a culturally acceptable way. I suggest that when kung fu becomes part of one's everyday life, it links up to a constellation of related ways of being-in-the-world, which is helpful for both non-Chinese and diasporic Chinese practitioners seeking cultural fluency. In fact, I took it as quite a compliment when my emergent physical and linguistic skills prompted several consultants at Hong Luck to begin approvingly referring to me as "half-Chinese" or "white, but really Chinese."

I have mentioned how ideas from Taoist philosophy (daantihn, yin and yang) and dispositions from calligraphy inform kung fu practice, but I would like to re-emphasize that theory is no substitute for embodied knowledge achieved through training. For example, there is a senior Hong Luck member who runs his own club (with the elders' blessings) but who neither speaks nor reads Chinese. This advanced practitioner is of European Canadian heritage, and he did not achieve proficiency in kung fu from studying Chinese philosophy. At Hong Luck's anniversary banquet in 2009, he explained that he developed his martial arts prowess through years of intense training under Master Paul. My consultant had not taken an academic approach to martial arts, but he was nonetheless steeped in Chinese culture. For example, he has visited China, continues to eat Chinese food at home regularly, and enjoys Chinese films/television (with subtitles) in his leisure time, which shows just some of the ways that participation in martial arts can open a door to culture. Although this example demonstrates that it is possible to achieve an advanced level of kung fu proficiency through diligent practice and informal exposure to Chinese culture, I nonetheless found that focused study expedited the process for me.

In discussing Chinese-ness in kung fu, I am cautious about imposing exclusive, essential, or reified qualities to any cultural practice. There is a Chinese way of doing martial arts, but it cannot be monolithic. The horse stance, for example, is also found in Okinawan karate, which may show an influence from China but does not necessarily make it Chinese. There is also considerable variation within Chinese martial arts according to style, lineage, and practitioner, not to mention the diverse social contexts of a now global phenomenon. Language, philosophy, symbolism, and media all contribute to the discourses that construct kung fu, but these things do not over-determine the movement. Instead, they may be thought of as contributing to a way of being that is as much physical as it is intellectual and social. It is unfortunate that the plural of *habitus* is also *habitus* because it would be clearer (and more accurate) to speak of kung fu *habiti* or *habituses*. Similarly, Delamont and Stephens have noted that the individualized habitus of Brazilian capoeira practitioners in the United Kingdom is "both a state of mind and a bodily state of being" (2008: 59), involving the intersection of biological, biographical, social, and cultural influences on emergent dispositions.

Martial Artists Becoming Lion Dancers

Hong Luck students must first seek approval from an instructor before attending any classes other than beginner's kung fu. For those wishing to participate in lion dancing, having strong kung fu stances is particularly important because they are the foundation of all the choreography. Earning the privilege of attending other classes can take anywhere from a couple months, up to a year or more, depending on a student's previous experience in martial arts, initial fitness level, dedication to training, and raw talent. At the time I started my research with Hong Luck, there was no regular lion dance class on the schedule because the ad hoc members of the performance team were sufficiently experienced that they no longer held rehearsals, except before special or unusual events. When Quang deemed me ready for lion dance training, he agreed to let me join two other students in forming a new class to be taught by Noah, the lion dance team leader. We trained once per week for about two-and-a-half hours, but we also began participating in lion dance gigs and parades almost immediately as a form of on-the-job training.

The other members of my cohort and I had all joined Hong Luck around the same time. My classmates were both second-generation Chinese Canadian and said that they had an interest in lion dancing because of its importance to their cultural heritage. Mario was a university student in his early twenties who had already earned a black belt in karate before he started at Hong Luck but did not speak any Chinese. Luigi was an adolescent with natural athletic ability who spoke Cantonese at home.[7] Neither of them had any previous training in music or dance, which was not a prerequisite. After confirming our kung fu basics by asking what choreographed forms we knew

---

[7] The names Mario and Luigi are pseudonyms.

and looking at our stances, Noah gave us a brief introduction to the ritual function of lion dancing and then wasted no time in beginning our training.

The vehicle for learning the lion dance at Hong Luck is the "traditional" routine, which according to Noah "has been passed down from generation, to generation, to generation . . . basically forever" (pers. comm. 14 February 2014). A kung fu generation is approximately a decade, and the choreography is not as ancient as Noah claimed; an inactive Hong Luck member who came back for a visit later told us that the routine had only been created in the 1980s—albeit from an older stock of movements and rhythms. Notwithstanding the potential problems of using the word "tradition" here, I will stick with my consultants' terminology. The traditional routine we learned involves approximately twenty minutes' worth of choreography and has a tripartite narrative: lion looking for food, lion eating, and happy lion. During my research, I never saw the whole traditional routine performed in public, although I have seen Hong Luck videos from the 1990s when it was still being done in its entirety at anniversary banquets. A number of members have agreed that the whole thing seems too long for today's audiences, especially because of the amount of repetition that many find boring. Despite the repetition, there is a wide variety of rhythms and choreography, so the traditional routine acts as a repository for the sonic and kinetic vocabulary of Hong Luck's lion dance. To suit the needs of any given performance, shorter dances would be choreographed from recombined sections of the full routine.[8] While the whole traditional routine was no longer performed in public, it was still considered valuable to practise it in class; Hong Luck members positioned lion dance as a way of cross-training for fighting, so the length of the routine was good conditioning.[9] Although the specialization of modern cross-training methods might be a more efficient way of building strength and fitness, I can certainly vouch for lion dance as an extremely good workout. After I moved away from Toronto in 2016, David confirmed with the elders about the relatively recent origins of the routine, and he decided not to focus on it in class anymore. Nonetheless, the traditional routine was the backbone of lion dance training at Hong Luck for approximately thirty years, and it deserves respect.

[8] NB: set choreography is often preceded and/or followed by freestyle dancing where the lion(s) mingle with the audience.

[9] Modern lion-head construction, design, and materials are on the lighter side, especially for the Hoksan equipment used in competition. Most of Hong Luck's lion heads are mid-range in weight. Old-school lion heads were reputedly much heavier because they were larger and used a thick plaster, rather than papier-mâché.

A lion head weighs between three and twelve kilograms (five and twenty-five pounds), so doing a twenty-minute dance with one requires endurance. When lion dancers first start training, however, they do so empty-handed (i.e., without actually using a lion head), which helps to reduce the number of things they have to coordinate and literally lightens the load. There is enough work to be done in learning the footwork, miming the lion-head movements, remembering choreography, and recognizing rhythms. Once we had a basic foundation, Noah taught us simple drills with the lion head, which we practised as exercises until we were familiar enough with both choreography and manipulating the mask to do both at the same time.

Lion dance pedagogy follows the same general pattern as martial arts, except that movement is always done in relation to drum rhythms. Students first observe the teacher's demonstration and then try to mimic it. Once learners have the general shape, they enter a feedback loop with their teacher: practise a movement, get comments, refine the movement, get more comments, and so on. In lion dance class, the drum rhythms are introduced at the same time as the movement, but without being played on the drum; Noah would say the drum rhythms as a loose set of onomatopoeic vocables while demonstrating the steps. Eventually, we learned to say the vocables while lion dancing, building our familiarity with the rhythms and integrating them with movement.

Learning the percussion parts and lion movements at the same time engrains them in a multisensory way, so much so that they become a sort of gestalt, as will be discussed in the next chapter. Furthermore, the vocables facilitate communication by rendering drum rhythms as speech. Being able to speak percussion parts is useful for teaching as well as for choreographing performances, because Hong Luck does not use any form of written notation. Vocables also let Noah stay closer to us while teaching, rather than having to be behind the drum. Once we got the hang of a section, however, Noah would play it on the drum for us. Section by section, our teacher repeated the pedagogical cycle until we knew the full traditional routine, which took almost a year.

Not surprisingly, lion dance involves a lot of horse stance, and other scholars have remarked on the homology with kung fu footwork (Hu 1995; Liu 1981; Slovenz-Low 1994). I would like to clarify, however, that while all of the lower-body postures of the lion dance are found in Hong Luck's kung fu basics, the way of moving between stances is different. Generally speaking, the character of the lion is meant to be powerful and fierce, yet also lively and noble. Novice dancers must continue to be able to stand strong, as they have practised in the beginner martial arts class, but they also learn to step more lightly and in a slightly exaggerated way that adds an aesthetic quality to the combative footwork.

A wide horse stance is important not only for physical stability, but also because it places dancers' feet past the edge of the lion's body, thereby making the legs look more balanced relative to the size of the costume. As one senior member was fond of reminding us, a tall and narrow stance makes the lion head look like a "goldfish on a stick." A wide horse stance takes up more space and gives the lion a stronger presence. My two main teachers and the other members of my cohort were all of less-than-average height in Canada (between 5'4" and 5'6" or 162–167 cm), but closer to normal in Southern China, which is the land of both their ancestors and the lion dance. Thus, they could sometimes get away with what Noah acknowledged was cheating by putting their feet wide apart without actually sinking too deeply into their horse stances. At 5'10" or 178 cm, I am a bit taller than average, so I had the extra burden of having to keep a lower stance as well as hunching my torso forward in order to keep the lion from looking too tall for the normative standard. A former lion dancer, who was a head taller than I, told me that he stopped performing because the ultra-deep stance and hunched body required of him were too taxing. Early on in training, the physical demands of maintaining a normative lion height felt like a handicap for me because it made everything more tiring. In the end, however, my body grew accustomed to it, which improved not only my dancing, but also my kung fu. I have grown to be comfortable in this deep, wide stance and, in the process, was forced to develop extra strength, endurance, and efficiency, which often come in handy in situations where cheating is not an option. Luigi, on the other hand, was still growing when we trained together, and he began to struggle with the lion dance body position required of him as his height increased. His foundation did not receive enough attention when he was shorter, which was exacerbated because he eventually gave up martial arts training in favour of lion dancing.

The way the upper body moves may at first appear to be dissimilar between kung fu and lion dance because of the mask, but there is a common quality. Hong Luck's characteristic lion movement is aggressive-looking because of its explosiveness, which draws on a martial habitus to execute what Noah calls *popping*. Dancers use short, punch-like gestures that shoot the head forwards, slamming the back of the mask into the neck and shoulders, before swiftly re-chambering and shooting the head again. As a result, dancers end up with scratches and bruises across their shoulders, despite the padding built into the lion head. Popping typically occurs during the walking sections of a dance, and it gives the appearance of a wild animal scanning the area. The violence of this movement brings the lion to life by causing its fur, eyes, and pompoms to shake. To inspire us, Noah told stories about one of Hong Luck's top lion dancers from a previous generation who earned the nickname "Guns" after a performance where his jerking/popping actually destroyed the mask with its vigour. Similarly, David referred to shaking the mask during head-up as *jerking*. He taught us to alternate punching one hand out while chambering the other in order to vigorously jerk the mask in the air, which draws on striking skills from kung fu. The level of aggression embodied in this style of lion dance is a distinctive specialty of Hong Luck and brings a martial flavour to performance that is often lacking in other groups, especially those who do not practise kung fu (i.e., competition lion dancers).

Lion dance draws on not only the physical stances and martial dispositions of kung fu, but also the synchronization skills implicit in the beginner class. For some Hong Luck students, training at the club is their first exposure to musicking and dancing. Following the teacher's counting in beginner kung fu class therefore functions as basic training in not only martial arts, but also timing. The importance of synchronizing to martial sound in beginner class was illuminated in the winter of 2013 when a new student, whom I will call Theodore, tried to join the lion dance class. Quang had approved his stances, but Theodore was apparently still having difficulty with basic synching. David had taken over for Noah by that point and was teaching the lion dance class. Theodore seemed unable to adequately match the timing of his movements to the vocables, much to our teacher's chagrin. This synchronization problem was evident right from the beginning of the traditional routine, where the lion is supposed to look around while blinking its eyes and chomping the mouth in time with a simple, even, accelerating pulse played on the drum. David had me demonstrate the movement while he said the vocables, then told Theodore to mimic me. Try as he might, Theodore could not match the empty-hand lion gestures to the rhythm. I attempted to help by exaggerating my movements, which mime the way one hand pulls a string in the mask to make the eyes blink, while the other hand operates the hinged mouth in opening and closing. David said the accelerating pulse rhythm again with increased enunciation, "Chek. Doooom chek. Dooom

chek. Doom chek. Dom chek. Chek. Chk, chk-ck-kk," but Theodore continued to move haphazardly and seemingly without regard for the beat.
After class, David told me that this would-be lion dance apprentice was not
ready and needed to go back to beginner kung fu class for remedial training.
I asked why, considering that Theodore had an excellent horse stance. Was
moving in time with the beat a kung fu skill, rather than a question of dance
ability or musicianship? David replied exasperatedly, as though it were self-
evident, "YES!"

Lion Dancers Becoming Percussionists

As my classmates and I learned the traditional lion dance routine, we
also started to play the percussion, beginning with the accompanying
instruments. We started with cymbals almost immediately, as do all novices,
because they are the easiest instrument, in terms of both technique and
rhythm. In class, it also made sense to start everyone on cymbals so we could
play together; in a standard lion dance gong and drum ensemble, there is only
one drummer and one gong player, but if there is a surplus of performers, additional percussionists take up a set of cymbals.[10] At Hong Luck, it would be
rare to have more than four people playing cymbals in a performance, with
one or two cymbalists being most common.

Cymbal playing emerges from the basic synchronization ability developed
in kung fu beginner class. Our first lesson from Noah was to simply follow
the beat of the drum. By the word *beat*, he meant the underlying pulse of the
tempo, so we started by playing a steady stream of quarter notes. Next, Noah
told us to stop when he stopped and to keep our eyes on him as we played
so that we would know when to stop. At that point, the drum rhythms were
still unfamiliar, but Noah's body language provided clues as to where there
would be rests and when he would stop. He would make eye contact ahead
of pauses, as well as slightly exaggerate the final drum-stroke by raising his
hand extra high and then dropping lower into his stance on the last beat.
Once we could follow the basic beat, we learned to reserve quarter notes for
walking rhythms and to switch to a repeating motif of quarter followed by
two eighths for the head-up beat. Noah also taught us to match the drum

[10] The only exception to this that I have observed came during Hong Luck's fiftieth-anniversary
banquet, when a tiny handheld gong was brought out from storage to complement the usual
hanging gong.

rhythm—albeit more simply—in certain places, such as the three-rises. It was not long before I got to play the gong, too, although my classmates were a bit slower to progress, perhaps because of their lack of previous musical training.

The gong and cymbal parts are both subordinate to the drum, but their roles in the ensemble are slightly different. Cymbals basically fill out the soundscape because of their washy, ringing sound. The gong, however, accentuates the onset of each beat, particularly when performers use a stac-cato style. The gong rhythms are the same as those of the cymbals for the head-up and three-rises, but during walking, the gong player typically uses a counter-rhythm that interlocks with the drum pattern, consisting of: quarter rest, two eighths, quarter rest, and quarter note. The transcription in Figure 4.4 illustrates how the three instrumental parts fit together in repeating sections of the basic walking and head-up rhythms.

Because the gong part is not doubled, gong players have more room for variation than do cymbalists. David, for example, uses a couple of dif-ferent syncopated rhythms on the gong that resemble the timelines of West

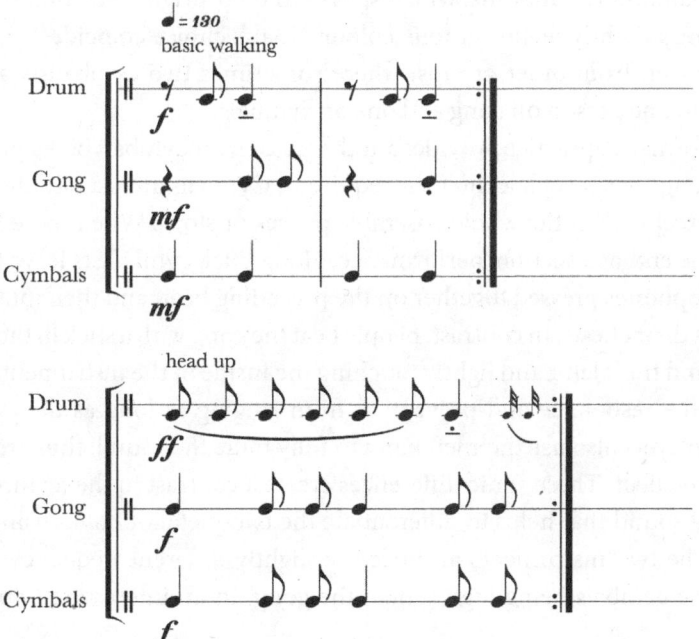

Figure 4.4 Transcription of ensemble walking and head-up loops
Credits: Colin P. McGuire

African bell patterns or the Afro-Cuban *clave*. There was only one other senior member who played more complex gong patterns, but, unfortunately, he was not very active during my fieldwork. When I asked David about the origin of his timeline-esque gong patterns, he vaguely said he had heard them somewhere. Later, he pointed me towards the YouTube channel of a group in Hong Kong whose rhythms had inspired him. In the Hong Kong examples, the timeline is played in unison on both gong and cymbals.[11] Generally speaking, rhythmically complex patterns are uncommon for the accompanying instruments in traditional Futsan lion dance percussion, although they seem to be gaining popularity among more contemporary-minded groups. Anecdotal testimony from a senior Hong Luck member suggests that these timeline patterns may have been introduced into the repertoire by Chinese migrants who had spent time in Cuba, though I have not been able to confirm this claim.

Whereas the gong allows more rhythmic freedom, the cymbals are a more essential component of the ensemble's sonic texture. I discovered this hierarchy when we were shorthanded for a gig one night and Noah had to choose between cymbals or gong. He opted for cymbals, explaining that they are louder and more sonorous, which speaks to their bright, rich timbre versus the gong's slightly mellower tone colour. Noah's choice coincides with what I have seen from other groups, where sometimes two cymbalists are preferred to one person on gong and one on cymbals.

Performance practice provides another reason for cymbals being preferred over gong (when such a choice is required). Cymbals are usually allowed to ring, except when the whole ensemble pauses or stops. When there is a rest or at the end of a section/performance, Hong Luck cymbalists leave the two metallophones pressed together on the preceding beat, and then mute them against their chests. In contrast, people beat the gong with a stick in their right hand and their left hand lightly touching the inside of the instrument, which stifles the resonance and prevents it from ringing as long as the cymbals. Gong players also use their left hand to fully mute the sound, thus creating a staccato effect. These sonic differences create a contrast in the texture of the martial sound that helps to differentiate the two metallophones using duration. The two instruments also occupy slightly different frequency ranges, with the cymbals being higher than the gong. In an interesting opposition

---

[11] http://youtu.be/9iaPxsHu2_E?t=2m5s.

to the typical hierarchy of many types of music, the lowest-frequency instrument in the ensemble, the drum, is the main or lead part.

The Practical Logic of Drumming

Frank Ng [Ǹgh Hóng, 吳宏] is Hong Luck's master drummer, but he no longer regularly participates in training or performances due to the onset of Parkinson's disease. At the club's fiftieth anniversary in 2011, he shuffled into the club in the morning with shaking hands and a slightly slack mouth, so no one expected him to do any drumming. However, when he stood in front of Guan Yu's altar and picked up the drumsticks to play for the first lion dance of the day, he was transformed from a weak, old man to a powerful martial sound artist. His performance was authoritative and seemed to come from somewhere deep within him that had remained impervious to the ravages of disease. It may not have been as loud or as fast as it used to be, but Frank nonetheless held forth masterfully, humbling most of the club's younger drummers.

At the banquet that evening, I had the opportunity to sit next to Frank, which was a rare opportunity to soak up some of his wisdom. In conversation, I asked him about his martial arts and drumming background. He replied that he only began practising kung fu at Hong Luck when he came to Canada at the age of eighteen. Nonetheless, he explained that, before he left China, he had been immersed in lion dance culture as a youth in his native Taishan village for as long as he could remember. David was sitting on the other side of the large, round, communal table and asked Frank for some pointers on drumming. First, the master drummer humbly remarked that he had nothing to teach David, acknowledging the younger man's tremendous skill. Frank then qualified his response by neatly summing up the traditional approach to learning kung fu and lion dance drumming: "Everyone plays different . . . (you) hear it in everyday life and then just play it. Just play your life." An individual repertoire of rhythmic variations and the ability to embellish them are acquired slowly over time, requiring the personal appropriation alluded to by Frank.

For those not yet steeped in martial sound, figuring out what to practise on the drum is the first challenge—particularly because everyone is expected to play differently. In the spring of 2009, we had been having lion dance class for six months or so, and Noah decided to let us try drumming. It was a disaster. I suspect that Mario, Luigi, and I failed so miserably because we lacked sufficient experience to have fully embodied the rhythms. Noah helped us out by demonstrating a basic walking beat, which we repeated *ad nauseum* in a very uncharacteristic way (i.e., everyone the same and without variation). Three-quarters of our lion class was still spent dancing, but the last part was henceforth reserved for working on the instruments. Mostly we played cymbals and gong while Noah played the drum; it would be another half year before anybody's drumming would make any real progress. In the meantime, we played the drum infrequently in class, practising whatever we could remember or figure out for ourselves.

By the fall of 2009, my classmates and I had been lion dancing for almost a year and had nearly finished learning the traditional routine, so we were much more comfortable with the beats. Noah left for university, and David, who had much more virtuosic drumming skills, was teaching the class. By dint of having been more fully immersed in the rhythms, my cohort's first faltering attempts at drumming had unsystematically progressed to the point where we could hack out of some basic beats. This was truer of Luigi and I, because Mario showed little interest in—or aptitude for—drumming. For some of the specific rhythms in the traditional routine, the vocables make them abundantly clear and variation is minimal. Translating embodied knowledge into martial sound for such specific drum patterns was thus not too difficult. For other rhythms, however, variation and ornamentation are much more important, such as the walking beat or three-rises, which are common patterns for parades and performances. My classmates and I could play an approximation of the basic rhythms, but we were not doing it particularly well. In fact, David found our skills to be in such a sorry state that he decided to help us, although he often protested that no one taught him and he did not know how to teach. Towards the end of class, we would all take turns dutifully pounding away on the drum as our teacher watched, listened, and corrected mistakes or gave advice.

As with many aspects of Chinese culture, there is a four-character idiom to cover the phenomenon of putting forward one's ideas, skills, or understandings in an effort to draw feedback, corrections, or further information from a more knowledgeable person. In the context of teaching and learning, "throw tiles collect jade" [*pāau jyūn yáhn yuhk*, 抛磚引玉] means doing or saying something in the hope of receiving guidance.[12] As

---

[12] This idiom can also be used in conversation to humbly refer to starting a dialogue with one's own small ideas in order to attract more insightful commentary from others. As a strategy for war or chess, it can mean making a gambit.

I progressed at Hong Luck, I discovered that this approach is used not only for learning to drum, but also for participation in the advanced kung fu class, where senior students practise and practise, until the master gets up from his chair at the back to scold them. In fact, the idea is so embedded that some senior members actually referenced the idiom in English by saying that they were "just throwing tiles" when they were looking for feedback or commenting that the head instructor had "given some nice jade" when they received coaching from him.

When we threw sonic tiles to earn David's drumming jade, his commentary often surrounded physical things, rather than strictly "musical" ones. In particular, our teacher made sure that we grounded our drumming in the centred strength of the horse stance and that we generated power in our beats using loose, flexible drum-strokes. These physical approaches to drumming were familiar because they embody the dispositions used in kung fu, further driving home that Hong Luck's percussion is meant to be martial sound. More specifically, David told us to sink into our horse stances as a means of transferring bodyweight into each drum-stroke, rather than relying on arm strength alone. Then, as with striking in kung fu, power was meant to flow through the drumstick until an abrupt concentration of force upon impact with the head of the drum. Other senior Hong Luck members have made similar comments about drumming, suggesting that "it's like punching" or even "you have to punch the drum." David has also made martial analogies with drumming. When he was teaching me a choreographed kung fu form where one wields a pair of swords, he told me to hold the weapons like a pair of drumsticks: gripping firmly (but not tightly) with the thumb, index, and middle fingers, while leaving the ring and pinkie fingers looser. Whether in drumming or swordplay, this hand position facilitates abrupt circular contraction around a fulcrum, thus amplifying force into a whipping snap.

To his credit, David attempted to expedite our learning process by showing us some rhythms, variations, and ornaments, though he also seemed somewhat conflicted about not being fully traditional with this pedagogical move. His choice was perhaps linked to the reasons my cohort had the opportunity to start lion dancing after only three months of basic training: Hong Luck was short of performers. At the same time, David sincerely wanted to help us learn, and he recognized the barriers imposed by leaving students to their own devices. Without entirely formalizing the transmission process, he facilitated our learning more than his teachers had done for him. I learned more about drumming from David than I did from anyone else, although I must reiterate that most of our class time was still spent on lion dancing.

During an exchange to Hong Kong in 2011–2012, I was able to do comparative observant-participation with the New Asia Kung Fu Society. On my first day of class with them, I was asked to demonstrate one of my Hong Luck forms so that they could evaluate my level. Satisfied that I had a decent horse stance and could do some kung fu, Master Joe Kwong asked me what I wanted to learn. Without hesitation, I replied drumming, to which he agreed. Nonetheless, he still wanted me to learn some of their kung fu first. After several weeks, Master Kwong finally asked me to play the drum for him so that he could evaluate my level. His comment focused on my ornaments, which were admittedly quite stiff. He suggested that it would help to practise them separately, and then he showed me how to loop triple and quintuple rolls as a rudiments exercise. Technique drills on the drum appear to be rare, however, and most drummers—at Hong Luck or at the New Asia Kung Fu Society—mostly try to play full rhythm patterns, working on beats, ornaments, and sequences all at the same time. I continued to play the drum whenever I could, hoping to attract more feedback. A couple months later, Master Kwong made a second comment about my drumming. He pointed out that I was subtly emphasizing the wrong beats, helping me realize I was unconsciously imposing a metric hierarchy that was not germane to Chinese martial percussion. I will return to this point in the next chapter, but suffice it to say that this pro tip literally turned my drumming around, because the strongest beat is the last one in a phrase, not the first.

When I returned to Hong Luck, I tried to play the drum whenever I could, which proved useful for collecting more feedback from the community of practice. Even when I practised before or after kung fu training, rather than during lion dance class, I soon discovered that senior members would offer comments or criticisms. Even people with little-to-no experience as drummers could still tell if something did not sound right based on their long experience with martial sound, which helped to intersubjectively evaluate my efforts. I was also lucky to receive coaching from some seniors who did know how to drum, but who did not attend lion dance class. One of my classmates, for example, had his own club and only came back to train at Hong Luck during the Sunday advanced session with Master Jim. This classmate gave me important tips about how to produce variations on the walking beat using ornaments, as well as insight into how these variants could be linked together in stylistically appropriate ways.

Due to the lack of a separate curriculum for drumming in kung fu clubs, instruction is unsystematic and practice is self-directed, which makes active membership in the community of practice essential. Haphazard pointers and tips come from a variety of people—if a learner continues to put themselves out there for criticism. My classmate Luigi was interested in drumming, but after his initial basic training in kung fu, he chose to only attend lion dance class, performances, and parades. He therefore did not regularly engage with the wider Hong Luck membership. As a result, he only received corrections from David and Noah, which slowed his progress compared to what he might otherwise have achieved. Learning to drum at a kung fu club is a social process. Although the lion dance teachers are important and hold authority, there is no simple instructor/learner dichotomy; instead, the whole group contributes to the transmission process.[13] In the next section, I delve into the relationships that structure a kung fu club as a social group in order to reflect on their distinctive qualities.

Pseudo-kinship and the Community of Practice

Full-fledged Hong Luck members contribute to the club physically, financially, and socially, earning their positions within the club's structure. It was not until I began bringing in revenue as a lion dancer and helping out with building maintenance that I became fully accepted as part of the group. My acceptance was also a function of having attended classes weekly for over a year; but helping out is what separates the core membership from regular students. Some kung fu students come to class and pay tuition but do not lion dance, play instruments, teach, or maintain the premises. While their tuition is important, on another level, they take more than they give. Some senior members do more teaching or performing than learning and thus are not required to pay tuition, but sometimes they pay anyway as a donation to the club. For me, being incorporated into Hong Luck on a deeper level meant that people were more willing to share resources and knowledge, which was helpful as both an apprentice and a researcher.

---

[13] This chapter is about what happens inside Hong Luck, but individual practice outside the club is also an indispensable part of learning to drum. David told us that we could—and should—practise anywhere by tapping out rhythms with our hands on any available surface, and Luigi and I both did this to positive effect.

The Chinese name for social connections came into English from Mandarin; "guanxi"[14] [*gwāanhaih*, 關係] means relationships built on trust, loyalty, and obligation. Basically, guanxi networks of mutual indebtedness bind people together through exchanges of social capital. This concept is an important part of familial, social, and business relationships in Chinese culture, so it is not surprising that it also governs many interactions at Hong Luck. Note that Guanxi can also have negative implications when these exchanges lead to bribery and corruption, which anthropologist Josephine Smart (2012) has identified as a growing problem in Mainland China.

An example of good guanxi at Hong Luck is being entrusted with a key to the building. These are in limited supply, and several senior members (at different times) have given me theirs on long-term loan, thus imparting the privilege of twenty-four-hour access to the martial hall and the responsibility to help out with teaching, lion dancing, and/or building maintenance. Good guanxi is also essential for learning how to drum, because the lack of formal instruction in drumming requires a prospective drummer to draw on many relationships in order to glean collective knowledge from the community of practice. Moreover, after so many years spent at Hong Luck, I now feel a visceral sense of obligation to the club. Guanxi relationships are built with favours, gifts, and goodwill to the point that the debts can never be repaid, which is how relations and connections become cemented.

Another way that a kung fu club builds relationships is through a social hierarchy based on pseudo-kinship. These ties of affinity are manifested in the titles that members use to refer to one another, which are always in Chinese, even when people are speaking English. These terms are based on familial relationships, and most of them are prefixed by the word for "teacher" [*sī*, 師].[15] My fellow students fell into one of four categories: "senior-classmate-sisters" [*sījé*, 師姐], "senior-classmate-brothers" [*sīhīng*, 師兄], "junior-classmate-sisters" [*sīmúi*, 師妹], and "junior-classmate-brothers" [*sīdái*, 師弟]. The head instructors were "masters" [*sīfú*, 師傅], but also "teacher-fathers" [*sīfú*, 師父], both of which are pronounced the same but written with different characters. Anyone could refer to a kung fu master (male or

---

[14] *Guanxi* is pronounced "gwaan-shee."

[15] Other Hong Luck elders or associates who were not active in the training hall were called by their given names followed by a respectful familial title like "junior uncle" [*sūk*, 叔] or "elder brother" [*gō*, 哥]. During my fieldwork, there was a dearth of female association members who did not practise kung fu or have another title, but they might have been "junior aunt" [*yìh*, 姨] or "elder sister" [*jé*, 姐]. In Chinese, these terms can also be polite forms of address more generally, as among acquaintances, friends, and associates.

female) by the former title, while only students would call their male teacher the latter.[16] To complicate matters, some of the senior members at Hong Luck were masters in their own rights, although within the club's hierarchy, they were still sije or sihing, rather than sifu. As far as I can tell, there is no female equivalent to the title sifu as teacher-father, although I have seen the term applied to kung fu masters who are women using the other way of writing it. At Hong Luck, the equivalent term, "teacher-mother" [sīmoú, 師母], was reserved for the head instructors' wives—even though neither of them practised kung fu. The pattern of male occupational nouns encompassing a supposedly "neutral" meaning is an example of how the Chinese language manifests gender (Ceccagno 2006:224, 227). In the final section of this chapter, I discuss several ways that gender is embodied in kung fu and lion dance.

Lion Dance and Gender

There are important distinctions to be made in the study of music in/as culture (among other topics) between biological sex as *male/female* and gender as *man/woman* (Koskoff 1987), not to mention intersex and transgender considerations, but the cis-gendered, hetero-normative environment at Hong Luck allows me, in the following discussion, to conflate the terms into a simplified binary of male/men/boys and female/women/girls. Traditionally, only males performed the lion dance, and Hong Luck used to limit females to playing the instruments. Needless to say, not being allowed to lion dance meant that women would have been hard pressed to learn drumming because of the transmission process I have just described. Eventually, the club eased formal restrictions on the gender of lion dance students, but women continued to face barriers thrown up by conservative senior members and patrons alike. During my fieldwork, most of Hong Luck's lion dance performers were still male, and there were no females who could play the drum well enough to do gigs or even parades. Interestingly, martial arts training has been much more inclusive, and, while men still dominate in

---

[16] Throughout this book, I have chosen to refer to Hong Luck's founders by the English honorific *master* because that is the club's practice when communicating with outsiders, particularly those who are non-Sinophones. Internally, however, Master Paul Chan and Master Jim Chan are typically referred to using the Cantonese word for master and their English given names, i.e., Sifu Paul and Sifu Jim (or Sifu Jin in romanized Taishanese).

terms of numbers, women have been performing Hong Luck's kung fu at a high level for decades.

In this section, I present ethnographic observations of the first females to perform the lion dance under Hong Luck's aegis. In contrast, some other Chinese lion dance teams that I observed in Toronto and Hong Kong have long been co-ed, and I note that all-female groups have been formed in other places to circumvent discrimination.[17] For comparison to Hong Luck's slower rate of change, I present ethnographic data from an interview with a senior member of the Ladies Lion Dance Team in Vancouver, BC. In the following section, I then deconstruct ritual justifications for the traditional exclusion of women, which reveals latent discourses of marginalized masculinity that are embodied in the lion dance. As philosopher Johanna Oskala has reasoned, phenomenologically accounting for gender requires understanding "how gendered experiences are constituted and how their constitution is tied not only to embodiment, but also to the normative cultural practices and structures of meaning" (2006: 240). She also argues that such reflection requires a critical distance from the experience, proposing that analysis of ethnographic or psychological data would be more appropriate than first-person phenomenology. Through examining sociocultural assumptions about Chinese masculinity, I seek to tease out some of the lion dance's gendered meanings, as well as examine how transgressive performances by women can reconstitute the embodiment of gender in empowering ways.

At Hong Luck's 2010 Chinese New Year parade, a group of lion dancers from an affiliated kung fu club came to help, including several girls in their early teens. Hong Luck members commented to me that it was unusual, and one long-time lion dancer told me that it was the first time he had ever seen a female do the lion dance. At that point, Hong Luck had no female lion dancers of its own. During the parade, I did not see any patrons preventing the girls from performing, but they probably assumed the female lion dancers were actually male. During parades, there are only brief moments when lion dancers' genders might be obvious, because performers are supposed to stay in character by keeping themselves covered by the lion head during performance and not removing it between performances. Additionally, winter clothing further obscures lion dancer's faces and bodies during Chinese New

---

[17] In North America, the leading all-female lion dance group is Gund Kwok [Gàn Gwok, 巾幗], who were formed in Boston, Massachusetts, in 1998, partially in response to the barriers women faced at traditional kung fu clubs. Unfortunately, I was unable to obtain an interview with them.

Year parades in Toronto, so the girls' gender identity was more concealed than it might have been in warmer weather. I did see some patrons looking distressed when they realized there were girls under the lion head, but that was only after the ritual had been completed and the girls were passing the heads to other performers.

In subsequent years, some patrons became more vigilant and made complaints to senior Hong Luck members about female lion dancers. During the fiftieth-anniversary parade in the summer of 2011, the same affiliated kung fu club from the 2010 New Year's parade came to help, and their group again included several girls. Hong Luck's anniversary celebrations are in August, so the warm summer weather meant that performers were more visible than they had been during the wintertime New Year's parade. Within the first hour of the anniversary parade, the girls were completely barred from lion dancing by Hong Luck's leaders after a storeowner was displeased with one of their performances. Near the beginning of the parade, a relatively inexperienced girl did a sloppy lion dance routine, which the receiving patron blamed on her gender. For the rest of the day, Hong Luck seniors enforced a proscription of female lion dancers, arguing that the girls were neither skilled enough, nor sufficiently strong. They further argued that the club's fiftieth birthday was a special event, so only more experienced lion dancers should perform, all of whom were male. Be that as it may, male lion dancers who lacked strength and/or experience were only prevented from doing more important performances, not barred completely. I surmise that the 2011 ban on females during the anniversary parade had more to do with gender than ability.

By the middle of 2012, a young woman named Bertha "Bee" Sun [*Syūn Wihng-sī*, 孫詠詩] was learning to lion dance at Hong Luck. She was my girlfriend at the time, and David recruited her to help with a last-minute gig where we did not have enough people. Luckily, she had a martial arts background and good enough stances to follow my lead footwork passably well from the lion tail. After that gig, David invited Bee to join the lion dance team, but he stipulated that she still needed to do a crash-course in Hong Luck's kung fu in order to familiarize her with the club's movement style.

During the Chinese New Year parade of 2013, gender discrimination against Bee was more transparent than in the first few years when girls from the affiliated club had started performing in Hong Luck's parades. Concerned patrons had grown wise to the possibility of females being under the lion and became vigilant about performers' gender. Some patrons were not fussed, but others started watching the dancers as much as the lions, complaining as soon as choreography revealed a glimpse of a female performer. Some patrons went further by pre-emptively requesting male lion dancers only. The fact that Hong Luck's leaders acquiesced to this pressure discouraged the club's lone female lion dancer, and she became ambivalent about participating in parades. Similar problems occurred at lion dance gigs, such as for store openings and weddings. Even if not all patrons excluded females, the rejection from those who did was hurtful—particularly when it was upheld by Hong Luck seniors. Furthermore, this barrier made it difficult for Bee to gain performance experience. While she continued to come to lion dance class and to help with gigs by playing tail or the accompanying instruments, her progress towards dancing the role of head was impeded.

Eventually, Bee was allowed to do formal gigs under the lion head—but not always without negotiation. Her first performance on stage did not happen until July 2014 at a banquet for the sixtieth anniversary of the Eastern Canada Taishan Association [*Tòihsāan Yāt Jūng Gā Dōng Haauhyáuh Wúi*, 台山一中加東校友會]. To the best of my knowledge, this was the first time a female had ever done a choreographed stage routine for Hong Luck. I also performed that night, along with three other lions (for a total of five), and I was relieved that there were no complaints about gender from the patrons or the venue. Given that it can be difficult to put together enough people for a five-lion performance, Hong Luck's seniors did not have the luxury of choice either. At the club's fifty-fourth anniversary in 2015, however, there was more debate about letting Bee do important performances—even though she was the most consistent student in the lion dance class, which I was teaching at the time. As she and I were preparing to do the initial performance in front of Guan Yu's altar to start the parade, several senior members came over to express concerns about the appropriateness of her gender for this important ritual. They suggested that Master Jim might not approve, to which I countered that we should let him decide for himself once he saw her dance. She and I assumed our positions next to the two lion heads on the ground and waited for Master Jim and Hong Luck's president to light incense at the altar. We then performed the first lion dance of the day in front of them, which they accepted. After we passed that hurdle, my seniors were more willing to let Bee perform the lion dance on stage at the banquet that evening, although they still expressed reservations about the ritual taboos. Their reticence suggested that perhaps it was not just Master Jim's opinion that they were worried about, but rather that they had their own stances on lion dance tradition and gender, too.

In comparison with Hong Luck, the Shao Lin Hung Gar Kung Fu Association [*Síulàhm Hùhng Kyùhn Gwokseuht Júngwúi*, 少林洪拳國術總會] in Vancouver, BC, has been more proactive about promoting gender equality in lion dance. Their group does a traditional style of Southern Chinese kung fu, and they have locations all over the lower mainland area. In 2004, Master Raymond Cheung [*Jēung Wáih-gwān Sīfú*, 張煒焜師傅] founded the Ladies Lion Dance Team in order to give women the opportunity to learn and perform. I interviewed Chiemi Fuse, who started studying under Master Cheung in 2008 and is now one of the lion team leaders. She very generously explained how their group has dealt with gender, the results of their untraditional approach, and her own experiences as an advanced lion dancer.

In our 2017 conversation, Chiemi told me Master Cheung was keen to teach anyone who wanted to learn, regardless of gender or ethnicity, but he also recognized potential barriers. All students at their club practise kung fu as well as lion dance and percussion, and the classes are co-ed. While the name Ladies Lion Dance Team suggests difference, Chiemi assured me that their training and performance practice is the same as that of their male classmates. Internally, the club avoids the potential for social awkwardness from mixed-sex physical contact by always pairing same-sex people under one lion, which was an issue I had not considered. When more females eventually joined the lion dance class at Hong Luck, people of both genders practised together. Bee did not mind co-ed dancing, but, in retrospect, there was some embarrassment from the other girl and the younger boys when it came to partner work that involved physical touch.

Apparently, the Shao Lin Hung Gar Association has sometimes faced criticism from other kung fu clubs as well as patrons. Master Cheung's commitment to equality led him to persevere, sometimes purposely sending the Ladies Team to important public events in order to make a high-profile point. His dedication eventually paid dividends. Chiemi recounted how she faced more scepticism in the early days, but that other masters have come to accept her and now include her in discussions about performances when several clubs do gigs together. She also said she has seen many patrons be pleasantly surprised when she takes off the mask after a performance and reveals her gender. Hard training and years of experience have forged advanced lion dance skills in her body, which allows her to performatively refute claims that women are somehow not strong enough to do it. Now, some patrons even request the Ladies Lion Dance Team, which gives Master Cheung's club a unique offering in the local market.

Sex discrimination in traditional Chinese lion dance raises the issue of socially constructed gender roles, but it does so in the relatively unexplored area of martial arts. The battle to overcome barriers to female participation has butted up against constructs that make gender limitations seem natural. As Judith Butler has so convincingly argued, gender is performed, "but if this continuous act is mistaken for a natural or linguistic given, power is relinquished to expand the cultural field bodily through subversive performances of various kinds" (1988: 531). Lion dance is an example of just such a subversive performance, as women resist and overturn limiting gender constructs. A contrasting approach would be mapping a different gender onto female biology, as described by Alejandra Martinez (2014) in her autoethnography of karate training in Argentina; she argues that her martial body is actually male. Rather than accepting martial arts as inherently gendered, Hong Luck's first female lion dancer rhetorically asked me, "why can't we just be lion dancers, not a woman lion dancer?" (Bertha Sun, pers. comm. 16 June 2017). Similarly, Chiemi explained that part of her motivation to get into martial arts was to embody strength as a woman, taking a stance on physical power that shows anyone can be powerful. In her own words:

> The thing was, since I'm . . . an Asian woman and pretty small, then a lot of, you know, people underestimate me, like you're so small, weak, you're just girl, and then I just didn't like that stereotypical . . . image. And then I really wanted to remove it, and also, I wanted to, kind of, present that I'm not that weak, can be strong. (Chiemi Fuse, pers. comm. 16 June 2017)

Despite advances in lion dance gender equality around the world, there remain vestigial reminders of difference even in more inclusive settings. For example, the Houston, Texas–based Teo Chew Association Unicorn, Dragon, and Lion Dance Team [*Chìuhjāu Wúihgún Kèihlèuhn Lùhng Sī Tyùhn*, 潮州會館麒麟龍獅團] won the inaugural United States Dragon and Lion Dance Championship in 2018 with a woman named Felicia Dang playing the head. The title on the trophy, however, was Lion Dance "King," showing a lingering gender bias. The Shao Lin Hung Gar Association's Ladies Lion Dance Team provides opportunities for women to demonstrate power through performance, thus empowering the performers, but it continues to do so in a marked category of gender by identifying the performers as "ladies." It will take time to fully overcome limiting preconceptions about lion dancers and gender, but at least progress is being made. I now turn to the traditional roots of gender taboos in lion dance.

Ritual Efficacy and Marginalized Masculinity

According to a Hong Luck elder named Uncle Wing,[18] "the lion dance disperses nefarious chi energy" [*móuhsī heui chèh hei*, 舞獅去邪氣] (pers. comm. 10 March 2013), which neatly encapsulates the ritual's logic and helps explain (though not excuse) the traditional exclusion of women. I wrote earlier in this chapter about the importance of embodying yin and yang through martial arts as a way of making kung fu more Chinese, and Taoist philosophy applies to lion dance, too. The yin principle is female, dark, negative, dead, cold, and associated with the moon, while yang is male, bright, positive, alive, hot, and associated with the sun; together they form the coextensive, mutually arising, and always-already-comingled nature of existence. In his discussion of martial arts and masculinity on the margins of Chinese society, anthropologist Avron Boretz notes that "the lion, it turns out, is a strongly *yang* creature with the power to drive away or destroy ghosts and other forms of death pollution" (italics in original, 2011: 54). My consultants rarely mentioned ghosts, but, as per Uncle Wing's explanation, they were adamant that lion dance should be strong and vigorous in order to be efficacious at getting rid of negative energy. In Taoist philosophy, female anatomy is fundamentally yin; a simple explanation for the exclusion of women is therefore that they have the wrong type of biological energy for the ritual.

A more nuanced hearing of lion dance in a kung fu context must take into account another culturally important binary: "civil and martial" [*màhnmóuh*, 文武]. The interleaved nature of yin and yang is reflected in a Chinese world-view that divides, organizes, and interprets society according to the civil jurisdiction of order, erudition, and refinement versus the martial realm of violence, strength, and action. According to East Asian studies scholar Krzysztof Gawlikowski (1987, 1988), the martial principle is yin because of associations with death, chaos, and destruction, although it functions by means of yang in the form of power, vigour, and bravery. This

---

[18] Uncle Wing's proper name was Chow Lin [*Jāu Lìhn*, 周練].

interpenetration is echoed in the civil principle, which is yang because it focuses on order, growth, and prosperity, although its virtues include yin qualities like peace, quietude, and introspection. Lion dance derives its yang power to expel yin energy from the strength of a martial foundation in kung fu, but the fighting skills that undergird the ritual are actually themselves yin because they are bodily tools for violent hand combat.

Chinese masculinity embodies the civil and martial dyad (Louie 2002), which provides a culturally embedded way of thinking about lion dance as a traditionally male practice that cuts across yin and yang. The archetypes of scholar and warrior, however, are not equally valued in Chinese culture; civil is the privileged category. For thousands of years, the Imperial Examination system determined who could enter the civil service and was thus a form of gatekeeping for social mobility. The exams changed over time, but their classic form extended from the Confucian tradition to cover areas like literature, poetry, law, ritual, and calligraphy. The high esteem of civil-ness persists to this day in Chinese culture, yet martial pursuits provide another path for men to achieve social status, particularly for those who do not fit the scholarly mould. Kung fu masters of the past, including Hong Luck's co-founders, rarely had formal education, and they relied on martial skill to overcome their deficit of civil acumen. Martial arts and martial rituals are therefore ways for marginalized males to actualize themselves in society as men (Boretz 2011; Dong 2016). Although these practices operate by means of violent yin energy, they require practitioners to embody yang ideals like strength, forbearance, and discipline. In particular, the yin martial violence of lion dance's ritual logic is transmuted in performance to become yang civil energy because it is generative, establishing order in liminal moments. Furthermore, the drumming's organizing effect adds to the civil qualities of the ritual—despite being martial sound—by providing clear structure to the performance. Beyond the ritual efficacy of martial yang driving away negative yin, strong lion dancing and powerful drumming can thus be socially transformative for men with little civil capital.

Notably, traditional Chinese stances on patriarchal hegemony took civil and martial to be wholly for men—not women (Louie 2002), which elides yin and yang considerations of female and male. The lion dance as community ritual was reserved for men to publicly showcase their masculinity through heroic displays of civil and martial virtue. My analysis is not meant to rationalize or justify the exclusion of women in Chinese culture, the worst example of which may have occurred in the PRC during the one-child-policy era (1979–2015), when families practiced female infanticide to insure that their single allowed offspring was male. Instead, my intention is to explain the socio-cultural context that made exclusively male lion dancing more meaningful for participants and audiences. The convergence of civil and martial in the lion dance transmuted strong yang energy into powerful social capital for marginalized men, which they had no interest in sharing with women.

Tying the ritual efficacy of lion dance to the gender of performers has problematic implications, not the least of which is naturalizing patriarchal social structures. If civil and martial are both the "natural" domain of men, then women are shut out and power becomes gendered. There is thus more at stake for women lion dancers than just performance opportunities. A senior Hong Luck member, who is herself a woman, told me repeatedly that men do the lion dancing because they are "naturally" stronger, more aggressive, and more dominant, which is required for the ritual. She was an advocate for maintaining the traditional exclusion of women, although she sometimes equivocated that she was being superstitious.

When Bee began to perform the lion dance for Hong Luck, it was an uphill battle to overcome gendered preconceptions with deep cultural roots. She was not just showing that women are capable of being yang, but also that they can command the power of both civil and martial spheres. With power comes responsibility, all the more so for a pioneer, which Bee remarked on thusly:

> Being the first girl under the head during . . . an anniversary performance on stage is, like, big shoes to fill, right? But also . . . you need to do that much better of a job onstage, cause otherwise if you slip up a little bit they'll be like, "oh, no, you're never allowed under the head again." (Bertha Sun, pers. comm. 16 June 2017)

In contrast to the traditional exclusion of women, non-Chinese male lion dancers and drummers have faced fewer barriers. In comparing our lion dance experiences as a Chinese Canadian female and European Canadian male, Bee commented that I might have faced scepticism, but that people were never angry—her gender had actually aroused their ire. On occasion, some patrons have certainly been sceptical of my ethnicity, and I have been condescendingly asked to my face if a "ghost fellow" [gwaílou, 鬼佬] like me actually knows how to lion dance, drum, or do kung fu.[19] Thankfully, such incidents were rare and only occurred a couple times in Toronto and once in Hong Kong. Notwithstanding Master Paul's exhortation to make my kung fu more Chinese, ethnicity does not appear to have been a problem at Hong Luck. Apparently, such acceptance was not always forthcoming from patrons in the 1960s and 1970s, and I have heard from some of my seniors that people occasionally tried to refuse non-Chinese lion dancers. Master Paul, however, did not yield to this pressure, maintaining a firm stance on promoting inter-cultural understanding through kung fu and lion dance. When I asked Master Jim for his thoughts on non-Chinese people doing kung fu, he inclusively said "Chinese people and Western people practising together is good" [Jūnggwok yàhn tùhng Sāi yàhn yātchàih lihn jauh hóu la, 中國人同西人一齊練就好喇] (pers. comm. 17 January 2016).

Conclusion

Drumming at Hong Luck emerges from familiarity with, ability in, and knowledge of kung fu as a blurred genre. According to the club's best drummers, they began playing more or less spontaneously after having been exposed to the percussion rhythms through long-term participation in martial arts and lion dance. My fieldwork experience confirms that there is no systematic approach to learning the drum, as compared to the more formal curriculum for kung fu and lion dance. The teaching and learning of music have received sustained interest from ethnomusicologists (Merriam 1964; Nettl 2005 [1983]; Wong 2004; Wrazen 2010), and Hong Luck's drumming falls under the category of what Timothy Rice (2003) calls *learned but not taught*. Prospective drummers embody other practices and transfer that embodied knowledge onto the drum. To be sure, elders, seniors, and peers provide tips, corrections, and commentary about drumming, so being an active part of the community of practice is important. Nonetheless, the route to becoming a drummer at the Hong Luck Kung Fu Club is still fraught. The path was laid out for me on the first day I walked into the martial hall, yet the journey to being able to perform was long, arduous, and complex. In this

---

[19] The Cantonese term *gwáilóu* [literally: ghost fellow, 鬼佬] is a reference to pale, "ghost-like," Western skin and can have somewhat pejorative connotations. A Western female would be a *gwáimūi* [literally: ghost girl, 鬼妹].

chapter I have described and interpreted my experiences of learning to drum through kung and lion dance at Hong Luck. As much as possible, I have also included observations of my cohort going through the same process, as well as lessons and ideas from our seniors and the elders.

While I have focused primarily on what happens inside the club, becoming a drummer does not end there. David suggested that my classmates and I should practise on our own time. He told us that he often uses his hands to play Hong Luck's rhythms on any available surface at home, at school, on public transit, and even at the dinner table. I began practising with my hands, too, and it eventually became a habit that I continue to this day. In a way, it has made martial sound a part of my everyday life, embedding the rhythms into the nooks and crannies of my being-in-the-world. Luigi also took David's advice and after a few months began to show a marked improvement in his coordination and timing. There are, of course, many differences between practising with one's hands on random surfaces and playing the big drum while surveying a situation and giving signals for a lion dance. Nonetheless, such practising constitutes an important aspect of the learning process.

To review, the broad strokes of Hong Luck's transmission sequence start with martial arts, progress to lion dance, add the metallophones, and finish with the drum, building layers of embodied knowledge that form a new kung fu habitus. My previous background in both music and martial arts gave me a running start, but it was still approximately five years before I was allowed to play the drum for performances. I am grateful to have had the time and opportunity to experience the traditional transmission process, and I argue that my embodied understanding is the richer for not having been fast-tracked. Kung fu basics establish a physical foundation through horse-stance training, centring practitioners in a Chinese way of being-in-the-world that is also the fundamental position for lion dance and drumming. As Master Paul taught me, kung fu forms need to look Chinese, which involves the expression of sensational cultural knowledge. I have identified a body-mind shift into the daantihn, embodying yin and yang energies, and flowing, calligraphy-like movement with a gathering acceleration of force, but there are surely others. In beginner class, students also become accustomed to following martial sound, synchronizing their strikes, blocks, and steps to the teacher's voice in a way that prepares them for lion dance class.

Apprentice lion dancers learn movement and rhythm together, embedding sound and movement in one step, which prepares people to become drummers. In class, we had to be able to say the vocables while simultaneously performing the dance, a challenge that helped engrain multimodal patterns of martial sound. Nonetheless, knowing the inter-media rhythms/movements and being able to perform them on a drum are not the same thing. The traditional routine we practised in class was an invariant set of choreography and percussion patterns, but performances require drummers to develop the ability to improvise rhythm and structure while leading the lion dancer(s), cymbalist, and gong player. To complicate matters, the drumming patterns used to accompany kung fu demonstrations are similar to lion dance rhythms, but they are not the same, and they are rarely heard at the club except around the time of the anniversary. Furthermore, good drummers need to develop their own way of playing, exceeding the basics of the tradition—without transgressing them—and adding elements of personal style. Despite the collective input of Hong Luck's community of practice, drumming is still learned, but not exactly taught, which makes it a prime example of the durability of a habitus and the economical transferability of its practical logic. In contrast to Bourdieu's classical idea of structuring structures inherited through lifelong socialization (1977 [1972], 1990 [1980]), a kung fu habitus is emergent and variable, particularly in a multicultural diasporic context that complicates simplex constructions of ethnicity. The dispositions engrained through training in lion dance and kung fu supply the necessary physical, musical, and cultural material for musicking with martial sound, but the results are variable and also highly personal.

Until recently, Hong Luck adhered to the tradition of excluding females from the lion dance ritual, highlighting the intersection of gender, performance, and embodiment in a Chinese martial context. During my fieldwork, I witnessed the first girls and women lion dancing with Hong Luck. Their performances were transgressive because they called into question both the rationale of yang ritual efficacy and the gendering of social power represented by male-only dancers. Female lion dancers, at Hong Luck and in other groups around the world, have shown that they are fully capable of delivering powerful lion dances, which belies the normative belief that girls/women are not "naturally" strong enough to do so. Despite the theoretically yin quality of their biology, females are fully able to embody yang energy in performance. Similarly, the civil and martial domains of society were traditionally reserved for men in Chinese culture, but women lion dancing to martial sound as way of bringing civil order to liminal moments challenges the perceived masculinity of these social realms. I wrote in Chapter 2 about how the lion dance was historically involved in resistance to oppression by the Qing Dynasty in China. I also detailed how it has empowered Chinese people in Canada facing institutional and social racism. An important part of the performance in both times and places has been for marginalized men to use kung fu as a way of carving out social space for themselves. It is not unique for there to be different meanings when women perform repertoire traditionally associated with men, as Caroline Bithell (2003) has observed in Corsican polyphonic singing. In the early twenty-first century, lion dance has evolved to include being a way of resisting limiting gender constructs through public community performances.

Now that I have explained Hong Luck's transmission processes for drumming, as well as some of the issues around embodying kung fu and lion dance, I can proceed in the next chapter to discuss the experience of martial sound. This chapter has described how practitioners come to embody a Chinese way of being-in-the-world with sound through kung fu, lion dance, and percussion, which notably transcends gender and ethnicity, while still being complicated by them. The kung fu method of learning rhythm follows Greg Downey's suggestion that in Brazilian capoeira "[d]ancing . . . is an apprenticeship in hearing" (2002: 504), as practitioners in both arts engage with martial sound through movement. I now direct my attention to how kung fu adepts hear with their bodies, as well as delve more deeply into the rhythm of combat.

5

Martial Sound in Motion

Choreomusical Meanings in Lion
Dance and Hand Combat

During Chinese New Year 2013, Hong Luck's lion dance team performed at
the Topcliff Public School in Toronto's north end, where we received a rock-
star-worthy reception. The teacher who coordinated the performance told
us that most of the students had never seen a lion dance before, but that they
had been introduced to Chinese New Year customs in their classes. When
we were ready to start, I poked my head into the gymnasium and noted that
it was packed with students sitting on the floor, waiting impatiently. Luckily,
there was a narrow pathway for us that went from the door through the
middle of the gym and ended at a small open space on the far end where we
could perform our routine. I was playing lion head that day and was amazed
at the sheer loudness of the children's reaction when we made our entrance;
the students of Topcliff briefly overpowered the percussion instruments
with their cries of excitement, yells of amazement, and, particularly from
the youngest ones, screams of fright. Many of the children were vigorously
waving small lion-head decorations, which they had made by colouring
paper stencils with crayons and affixing them to plastic straws. Their reaction was remarkable, and they were one of the most appreciative and demon-
strative audiences I had ever experienced as a musician, dancer, or martial
artist.

After the performance, the lion dance team returned to Chinatown for
our customary post-gig meal together, during which I remarked on the raucous reception we had received. Noah agreed that the children's enthusiasm
was impressive, but he dismissed it as being due to the novelty of the performance. Moreover, Hong Luck's lion dance team leader thought that the
kids did not truly understand what was happening and thus could not really appreciate it. Granted, very few of the students were of Chinese heritage,
but they had at least been introduced to New Year's lion dance traditions in
class, so I wondered what they were missing. I followed up by asking who are

Martial Sound. Colin P. McGuire, Oxford University Press. © Oxford University Press 2024.
DOI: 10.1093/oso/9780197775936.003.0005

the best, most appreciative audiences. Noah suggested that most people, including the students at Topcliff, only get a partial understanding of the lion dance because they hear the percussion only as "noise," but that practitioners actually know what the rhythms mean. After a moment of thought, Noah acknowledged that older folks who have a lifetime of experience with lion dance often have a good understanding, too. He then explained that the meanings he was referring to lay in knowing how lion dancing and percussion rhythms work together, which allows people to follow the performance even when they cannot see the dancer(s) clearly. As I discovered later in my fieldwork, Noah was not alone in hearing significance at the interface between sonic and kinetic; Master Jim taught a four-part way of understanding lion dance as the confluence of audile and motile factors.

In this chapter, I investigate meanings in kung fu's blurred genre (including martial arts, lion dance, and percussion) that can be found in the relationships between sound and movement. Ethnomusicologists have long taken an interest in dance, particularly because some cultures treat it as an integral part of music and vice versa (Chernoff 1979). For similar reasons, ethnochoreologists have attended to music (Kaeppler 2001), and both groups share an anthropological concern for socio-cultural context. Nonetheless, in keeping with the central concerns of the respective disciplines, most ethnomusicologists privilege music, while ethnochoreologists tend to focus on dance. In the 1990s, however, scholars interested by music and dance in equal measure began to focus on the relationships between them, thinking in terms of choreomusicology. At first, work in this hybrid area sought to bridge the gap between Western art music and concert dance (Hodgins 1992; Fogelsanger and Afanador 2006; Jordan 2011), but anthropologist Paul Mason (2014) has shown how a choreomusical perspective can be useful for studying expressive culture from other places, too. Notably, Mason (2016a, 2016b, 2016c, 2017) has engaged with both Indonesian pencak silat and Brazilian capoeira as blurred genres of martial arts that include music and dance. In his helpful article summarizing, adapting, and extending the approaches of choreomusicology, we see/hear how humanly organized sound and humanly organized movement (note the broad characterizations) can be studied according to "[t]he direction of choreomusical relationships, the intrinsic interactions and the extrinsic connections," which "are all a result of creative processes, artistic collaborations and aesthetic preferences within social and cultural contexts" (Mason 2012: 21). In a framework adapted from Paul Hodgins (1992), Mason lists intrinsic interactions as rhythmic, dynamic, textural, structural, qualitative, and mimetic, while grouping extrinsic ones as archetypal, emotional, and narrative (2012: 18). Building on this body of literature, my work on martial sound looks at—and listens to—how people take a stance on directions, relations, interactions, and connections between the sonic and kinetic in order to (re)construct meanings in experience.

This chapter is structured as follows. I start with a philosophical consideration of embodied cognition, focusing on the fundamental schemata most relevant to my interpretation of martial sound. Next, I delve into Master Jim's ideas about the meaning of lion dance at the juncture of percussion and movement. Then I extend the choreomusical method to investigate how martial sound can help make hand combat more intelligible through musical rhythm. In accordance with the plan I laid out in the book's Introduction, I am continuing to tighten the focus from the broad and external to the narrow and internal. The chapters on social history, public performance, and private training have established a contextual foundation. Now it is time for me to delve into the corporeal cognition of martial sound.

The Entrainment Schema and Cognitive Metaphor

My fieldwork consultants consistently emphasized embodied knowledge as the key to understanding their martial sound, which suggests an epistemological problem for non-practitioners. Drawing on distinctions between the understandings of insider versus outsider, Clifford Geertz problematized ethnographers trying to study people's experiences when he wrote,

> The ethnographer does not, and, in my opinion, largely cannot, perceive what his informants perceive. What he perceives, and that uncertainly enough, is what they perceive "with"—or "by means of," or "through"... or whatever the word should be. (1983: 58)

My solution as a researcher has been to follow my consultants' advice and become a practitioner, bringing me as close as possible to their perspective in order to arrive at a hybrid insider/outside understanding (Rice 1994). To produce an ethnography, however, requires explanation suitable for non-practitioners. In his study of listening in Brazilian capoeira, Greg Downey cites Geertz as inspiration to focus not on what capoeira adepts hear in their music, but rather what they hear with, by means of, or through, that is, the skilled body (2002: 288). In addition to explaining how adepts perceive their martial sound, I propose that embodiment theory offers generalizable modes of cognition that are available to non-practitioners and can provide readers with insight into unfamiliar bodily practices.

Scholarly interest in the body as a site of sense, logic, and significance has been growing steadily for quite some time. Although research on embodiment in the humanities and social sciences is not new (e.g., Mauss 1934; Merleau-Ponty 2002 [1942]), it has been gaining increasing prominence in recent years. Historically slow growth in this area can be at least partially attributed to the dominance of Cartesian dualism in Western thought, but many scholars have become critical of oppositions that pit body against mind, emotion against reason, and subject against object (Csordas 1990; Johnson 1987; Walker 2000). Briefly, the philosophical tradition of René Descartes privileges a carefully constructed objectivism where abstract thinking as expressed in propositional language is the only "true" reality. By extension, embodied knowledge, lived experience, and subjective intentionality are classed as "inferior." In Buddhist philosophy, however, the discursive intellect (i.e., the mind) is one of the six senses, along with vision, taste, touch, smell, and hearing, and is therefore not separable from the subjectivities of the body (Kapleau 1965: 13, 101). This non-dualism is important for Hong Luck, with its kung fu tradition being linked to Buddhism through Shaolin Temple mythology; and my consultants have consistently directed my research back to physical praxis as the path to understanding.

As Margaret Walker remarks, "some of the clearest support for an embodied theory of music cognition and meaning comes not from musicologists, music philosophers or psychologists, but from dance scholars" (2000: 38). One of the finest examples of such scholarship is Tomie Hahn's (2007) work on transmission in Japanese dance. Nonetheless, I should point out that, notwithstanding the dance orientation of her book, Hahn is trained as an ethnomusicologist. Other music scholars who engage deeply with dance as part of their research are also making important contributions to embodiment studies (Friedson 1996; Rahaim 2012; Wrazen 2010). In a paper on terminology in music and dance, Jörgen Torp (2013) has suggested that it would make sense to use common terms that apply to both, pointing to the importance of choreomusical relationships. My concept of martial sound expands from that idea by providing a way for musical vocabulary to be used in fighting arts, where practitioners, teachers, performers, coaches, and athletes rarely have the terminology that dancers might have to discuss their embodied being-in-time.

Anthropologist Thomas Csordas (1990) collapses the Cartesian dichotomy by grounding the existence of culture in the body. To do so he draws on Merleau-Ponty's concept of pre-objective (but not pre-cultural) perception and on Bourdieu's logic of practice as embodied in the habitus. In this way of thinking, the body takes its place as the root of culture because it determines how—and thereby what—we perceive, and our perception is, of course, always already shaped by our existence as social beings. In a parallel vein, philosopher Mark Johnson locates the cognitive ground of culture in the body (1987), and he has applied this theory specifically to music (1997). Johnson's work on embodied cognition has been cited favourably by a number of music scholars (McClary 1994; Rice 2003; Zbikowski 2004), and it has been used as the basis for extended analysis by others (Echard 1999; Walser 1991).

In Johnson's cognitive semantics, the body is the basis of culture because it provides the primary experiences of meaning that support processes of perception, judgment, and reasoning. From this perspective, he argues that the body is in the mind. Johnson calls the primary categories of embodied knowledge *image schemata*, which are pre-linguistic, pre-conceptual structures that connect—and give meaning—to a host of similar experiences. A schema is necessarily abstract and general so it can be attached to other more concrete and specific aspects of existence through metaphor. Used in this way, the word *metaphor* is not intended in the rhetorical or literary sense, but rather as a fundamental way of understanding one area of experience through another. This type of metaphorical approach is also found in Steven Feld's (1990) work on the articulation of social identity through musical aesthetics among Kaluli people and John Miller Chernoff's (1979) linkage between rhythmic music and social values in West Africa. Johnson explains:

in order for us to have meaningful, connected experiences that we can comprehend and reason about, there must be pattern and order to our actions, perceptions, and conceptions. *A schema is a recurrent pattern, shape, and regularity in, or of, these ongoing ordering activities.* These patterns emerge as meaningful structures for us chiefly at the level of our bodily

movements through space, our manipulation of objects, and our perceptual interactions. (italics in original, 1987: 29)

One of Johnson's main examples is what he calls the *force schema*, which has
a number of gestalt structures arising from it. An understanding of force is
basic to navigating gravity, locomotion, and object manipulation, among
many other things. On higher cognitive levels, the force schema allows us to
understand how an airplane can be propelled by its jets, as well as how social
pressure can compel someone to join the local Parent/Teacher Association
(Johnson 1987: 2). Robert Walser (1991) provides an excellent summary of
Johnson's thinking, as well as an example of how one might apply the force
schema to music by interpreting perceptions of power in the overdrive of
heavy-metal guitar distortion.

The unexplored image schema most choreomusically relevant to martial sound is what I propose to label *entrainment*: "a phenomenon in which
two or more independent rhythmic processes synchronize with each other"
(Clayton, Sager, and Will 2004: 1–2). The preceding definition includes the
caveat that one system of vibration must not be directly created by the other,
as in the case of resonance. Another definition leaves room for agency or variation by emphasizing the role of perception and response, rather than pas-
sive synchronization: "spatiotemporal coordination resulting from rhythmic
responsiveness to a perceived rhythmic signal" (Phillips-Silver, Aktipis, and
Bryant 2010: 3). The second, broader entrainment framework is important
for martial sound because the authors extend it to include non-pulse-based
rhythms, such as language and gesture. Hand combat is often rhythmic, but
it can lack the steady beat found in most styles of music. Nonetheless, entrainment is also important for musical significance because it grounds many
nonreferential meanings (Sager 2012: 32). More specifically, musical entrainment establishes being-in-time that negotiates and organizes relationships
through transcendent experience. These non-referential meanings thus do
not refer to specific objects or ideas, but rather use patterns of sound and
movement that "orient the person within time as well as within their physical
and social surrounding" (Sager 2012: 32).

I contend that the entrainment schema provides an ideal framework for
thinking about embodied choreomusical meaning in martial sound. It is
central to what practitioners perceive with, by means of, and through, but it is
broad enough to be available to non-practitioners, too. Further to Johnson's
cognitive semantics, entrainment undergirds not just nonreferential musical

meaning, but also a wide variety of lived experiences, which is what allows it to be a fully formed metaphor.[1] We experience it as babies when our caregivers sing or gently rock us to entrain our consciousnesses into sleep. Once we start learning to walk, we hold our caregivers' hands, and we must adjust our walking pace to keep up with them (and they to us). When we can walk on our own, and eventually run, we need to internally coordinate the rhythms of our upper and lower limbs. Daily cycles of sunlight entrain our circadian rhythms, the phases of the moon synchronize oceanic tides, and the changing seasons impact the pace of everyday life. People are also subject to mechanical entrainment from the relentless clocks that structure working life. Notably, asynchronicity is also experienced through entrainment, which is important for understanding hand combat through martial sound. Lion dance is a more familiar example because of synchronization between movement and sound; and this is where I begin my interpretation.

The Four Components of Lion Dance's Meaning

Shortly after Chinese New Year 2013, one of Hong Luck's senior teachers invited me to begin attending the Sunday afternoon advanced class taught by the head instructor. Master Paul had passed away the year before, so Master Jim had assumed responsibility for teaching the club's most senior and advanced students. I was surprised at how he laid out the lessons in a remarkably clear, concise, and rapid way. It certainly helped that the attendees were already at an advanced level, but there was also a sense of urgency from our aging master. Master Jim was keenly aware of his own mortality, and he told us that he had not passed on all his knowledge. Other members of the advanced class also noticed the sense of urgency: whereas Master Jim used to slowly teach one movement of a choreographed form at a time, often taking a year to go through a whole routine, we learned three hand forms and three weapon forms from him in the span of a mere year and a half.

---

[1] One of my first professors as an undergraduate, Steven Otto, introduced me to the idea of entrainment, expounding an extremely broad point of view. His metaphysical perspective positioned music as the sonic manifestation of cosmic order, and this has had a profound effect on me. Otto pointed to quantum physics, where everything in existence is thought to be made of energy and is thus in constant motion, from sub-atomic vibration to galactic oscillation. Understood in this way, harmony—as a universal ideal, not just a musical one—results from entrainment on levels from the subtle to the celestial.

The advanced class focused mostly on martial arts, especially choreographed forms, but, in the spring of 2013, Master Jim took David aside to scold him about his drumming. Luckily, Hong Luck's head instructor did not seem to mind me listening to what he had to say, and it was an excellent opportunity to observe percussion pedagogy on a more advanced level. Master Jim's sense of urgency was apparent here as well, and the other members of the advanced class commented on how rare it was to receive so much knowledge in such a short amount of time. He started by saying that David played the drum well, which was actually high praise considering that our demanding teacher rarely deemed anything to be better than barely okay. The brief moment of approval turned out to be a backhanded compliment, however, because it led swiftly to a reprimand for drumming too quickly and too fancily, thus making the beats hard to follow for both other percussionists and lion dancers. Master Jim said he would start teaching David some drumming, which turned out to be a series of short, weekly, semi-private lessons within the advanced kung fu class. I continued to observe these fifteen to thirty-minute sessions over a period of several months, and my respectful lurking was eventually rewarded when I was able to participate as a lion dancer, cymbalist, or gong player while David played the drum.

Advanced lion dance drumming lesson number one hung the meaning of performance on the integration of sound and movement. Master Jim started by explaining that the meaning of lion dance encompasses four components all working harmoniously together: vocables, lion movement, drumming, and emotion. He then went on to emphasize that a group effort is required to bring out the significance in performance, which is why it was a problem if David drummed in a way that was too difficult for others to follow. Significantly, there was no mention of ritual function or symbolism; the meaning was present in the choreomusical relationships, not in abstract linguistic constructions or extra-performative values. Working on martial sound in Hong Luck's advanced class was a return to basics but with a new layer of detail and nuance, which is characteristic of kung fu pedagogy at the club more generally. I had learned about all four components in lion dance class, but they had never been presented in such an integrated, coextensive way.

As one of my teachers, David had more experience with the four elements than I, but it was plain that he was still struggling with how they were meant to work together holistically. After the lesson, he and I discussed Master

Jim's four-part structure. We agreed that the link between movement and drum rhythms was fairly obvious, but that vocables were usually relegated to teaching, practising, and rehearsing—not to the meaning of performance. Furthermore, emotion in lion dance seemed to us to be related to choreography of ritual action, as opposed to choreomusical relationships. Over the next few months, the four parts would become clearer; not surprisingly this clarity came as a result of practice, not just explanation.

Master Jim focused his lessons on a "walking beat" [*hàhnglouh gú*, 行路 鼓], although it was not one with which David was familiar. In fact, none of the active membership knew this beat; apparently the students who had learned it in the past had not transmitted it. Stylistically, the rhythm patterns did not appear to be either Futsan- or Hoksan-style drumming, and Master Jim said he had learned them in his home village in Taishan, so David and I opted to refer to them descriptively as either Taishan beats or simply Master Jim's beats. Not only were the rhythms different, but so was the way of learning them. Rather than starting with lion choreography, David needed to learn the rhythms directly through sound. Master Jim spoke the vocables first, and David was expected to repeat them back exactly. Once the vocables were correct, Master Jim would play the beat on a drum and then have David play it back to him. Notably, there was an exact correlation between onomatopoeic words and drum sounds, as well as between spoken rhythms and those played on the drum, which differed from the loose vocables normally used in lion dance class or at gigs. This learning process was repeated piece by piece until the whole sequence was complete, consisting of three larger sections that were sub-divided into smaller phrases of unequal length. As but an observer to the lessons, I had to learn the vocable patterns silently, and I had to wait to try them on the drum. Nonetheless, the vocables were surprisingly catchy, and so I had no problem remembering them, which made it reasonable for me to translate them onto the drum on my own time.

Compared to the loose way that Hong Luck members use vocables in other contexts, Master Jim's expectation of exact alignment between nonlexical vocal sounds and drum beats is similar to the oral "drum texts" [*lòhgú gīng*, 鑼鼓經] of Chinese opera. Like drum vocables in other cultures, such as *solkattu* and *konnakol* in South Indian Carnatic music, Chinese drum text vocables are a mnemonic device and a way of setting patterns/compositions. They are also a means of communication, allowing practitioners to speak rhythms to each other. In the weekly lion dance class, or for verbal communication to organize choreography for a gig, Noah and David used only underdetermined sounds, particularly when vocalizing basic rhythms that they would always vary in performance. Master Jim's use of vocables, however, had a precision that is exclusive to a few patterns in the traditional lion dance routine. More specifically, he said *chek* for a rim click; *dong* for an open drum tone after a rim click (sometimes after a rest); *chang* for all other open drum tones; and *chit* for a mute. His vocables for rolls and ornaments included: *da-dl-ek* for a three-beat roll on the rim; *da-dl-a-dl-ek* for a five-beat roll on the rim; and *ch-ch-chang* for a three-beat roll on the drum head, with more *chs* added for five-beat or continuous rolls. While it may be possible to render these vocables in sound-loan Chinese characters, Master Jim only ever spoke them to us, and so I am leaving them as phonetic representations.

Vocables were familiar to David, and he picked up the rhythms quickly, but he appeared to struggle with the use of silence as part of a drum pattern. As I mentioned in Chapter 3 regarding generational differences, the younger drummers at Hong Luck all use a much tighter, more staccato style of playing than the elders. For example, David frequently uses his wrists or fingertips to touch the drumhead right after striking it in order to dampen the decay of individual drum-strokes. This style is especially evident in the way the younger generation plays walking beats; it allows for more clarity when playing complex rhythms and ornaments at fast tempos. Furthermore, when David did use mutes for certain traditional patterns, he was in the habit of combining a drum stroke with simultaneous dampening of the drumhead to create a specific tone, rather than using silence as part of the rhythm. Examples include laying a drumstick flat against the drumhead while striking it with the other stick to make a hybrid click/drum-stroke, slamming a drumstick down lengthwise on the drumhead to create a simultaneous mute on the drum-stroke, and striking the drumhead while pressing on it with the other hand to slightly raise the drum's tone while muting its resonance. Master Jim's *chit*, however, is the action of stopping a drum sound, referring to the cut-off of a previous drum-stroke's decay. It is not just a rest, but rather an active silencing that stops the sound of the drum directly on a beat by muting it with one's hand. Master Jim's walking beat uses *chit* only in specific places, letting the drum's sound resonate freely everywhere else. That is to say, mutes are not an optional element of style in Master Jim's drumming, but rather they are a structurally significant part of the rhythm patterns.

By identifying vocables as one of the lion dance's four components, Master Jim ascribed to them an important role that went beyond pedagogical, mnemonic, or communicative value. He held that the vocables should continually undergird both drumming and lion dancing, serving as a fundamental connection between them. The significance of this idea is that the vocal patterns are still meant to exist during performance—even though they are not actually spoken out loud. Thus conceptualized, oral drum texts serve as a unifying framework for variations on lion dance and drumming. As an intervention into David's fast and free performance style, Master Jim encouraged him to more firmly anchor his playing in the vocables. Our teacher further explained that drummers and lion dancers can have a degree of choreomusical independence in their sound and movement, but only as long as they share a common root in the tacit oral drum text. This meaning gives vocables vastly more importance as an integral part of performance that exceeds teaching, learning, and communication. As I will explain in the case studies of this chapter, cleaving to the oral drum text once saved me from a near disaster during a lion dance gig when David played a complex variation that I was not expecting—we stayed together in time through the unheard vocables.

After drumming and vocables, movement was the next aspect of Master Jim's lessons on lion dance's four components, but he spent little time focusing on movement independently. Our teacher continued to concentrate on David's drumming during the advanced class, so the commentary about lion dancing was mostly directed at me; by that point I was Hong Luck's most active lion dance performer. Master Jim told us that the lion must follow the drum rhythm, but that the two together combine to make what he called (in English), "ACTION!" Over the course of the drum lessons, he gave a few brief demonstrations where he said the vocables for his Taishan walking beats and mimed lion movements. He would then say the same rhythm pattern in different ways by modifying tempo, volume, and inflection, which he then matched with his empty-hand lion dancing. I already knew from lion dance class that dancers usually follow the drummer's rhythms as cues for choreography and ritual action, but the added nuance was to match movement quality to the drumming's intrinsic features, too. It is worth noting that in some parts of a choreographed routine, such as the eating section, the choreomusical direction shifts so that the drummer must follow the lion's action and match rhythmic responses to choreographic cues. Similarly, drummers may follow intrinsic cues from lion dancers, as when a vigorous dance performance requires extra sonic gusto in the form of volume and speed, or when a tired lion needs slower but heavier beats to keep them going. Regardless of who leads or follows choreography and emotion, lion dancers entrain to the drummer's tempo, which establishes a fundamental ground for other choreomusical connections.

Master Jim's discussion of lion dance in terms of its relationship to drumming was a natural prelude for his discussion of emotion, which was the final of the four components. When he first told us that the lion should exhibit "happiness-anger-sadness-joy" [*héi nouh ōi lohk*, 喜怒哀樂], David and I took it literally. We discussed the idea after class but had trouble understanding a sad lion outside the context of rarely seen funeral performances. Upon further research, I discovered that this four-character combination is actually an idiom encompassing the idea of emotions in general. Master Jim later clarified his meaning by linking it to kung fu performance. Just as a good martial arts demonstration requires full commitment to embodying combative energy, so too does a good lion dance need intentionality and intensity. While Hong Luck's lions are often aggressive, powerful, and vigorous when representing the club's spirit and/or performing ritual exorcisms, they can also be noble, respectful, playful, affectionate, rambunctious, mischievous, curious, cautious, happy, excited, hungry, full, tired, sleepy, and so on. Emotion in the context of lion dance thus means performing states of being, rather than just feelings or sentiments.

Not all possible lion dance emotions would be appropriate for the walking beats that Master Jim used as an example throughout David's drumming lessons, but the point is that the drummer and lion dancer(s) need to work together in a way that exceeds the ritual action and the choreography. The four-part lion dance scheme therefore explains how the different components of a performance synergise choreomusically on an intrinsic level in order to generate extrinsic meanings. At the intrinsic core are the first three elements: (1) vocables that set the basic rhythm patterns, (2) drumming that expresses the vocables in sound, and (3) lion dancing that manifests the vocables in movement. Variations by drummers and dancers are desirable because they add visual, physical, and sonic interest, but they must remain connected to the oral drum text, which places limits on how much personal flair performers may employ. Metaphorically, vocables are the bones, and performance is the flesh. The fourth component is extrinsic emotion, which results from the intrinsic interaction of the formal properties in drumming and dancing. To achieve emotional performances, drumming must animate and energize the lion dance, while dancing needs to complete the drumming by giving it visual and spatial form in movement. This deep cooperation is meant to add a layer of choreomusical meaning that brings the lion to life.

The four components were very clear, but I should clarify that Master Jim did not codify how specific combinations of them would result in particular emotions (or states of being). Instead, he stressed that lion dance should be emotional, which leaves room for interpretation by performers (and by informed audiences) based on perspective, knowledge, and context. As an example, a slow walking beat, played simply with little ornamentation, may have any of several connotations based on whether it occurs within the choreography of a routine or in a freestyle, unchoreographed moment. When such a moderately paced, low-intensity, walking beat is played before the eating section of a choreographed routine, it functions as a holding pattern that can be extended as a long as necessary. Drummers often need to play this way when, for whatever reason, a patron is not quite ready to feed the lion; mellow walking keeps the performance going but creates a lull before the climax. In this context, lion dancers would usually interpret the beat as a cue for hungry choreography and start looking for food, but they might do so cautiously, tiredly, impatiently, mischievously, and so on. If, however, a relaxed walking beat was played after a banquet performance when the lion(s) mingle with the audience, the dancers could choose to interact using a variety of action-emotions: playful, affectionate, naughty, curious, aloof, and so on. In either case, lion dancers would still be following the rhythm established by the vocables and actualized by the drummer, while having some freedom in terms of the emotional quality with which they would perform.

Transcription of Lion Dance's Four Components

As a visual aid to help explain Master Jim's four-part lion dance scheme, Figure 5.1 provides an inter-media transcription for a walking beat. With all due respect for Master Jim's rhythms, I have selected a Futsan-style rhythm pattern, because it is much more typical of both Hong Luck's performance practice and kung fu lion dancing more generally. In terms of the fourth element (emotional content), this example is marked as *aggressively prowling*, but, again, similar rhythms and movement patterns could embody other emotions depending on the intrinsic qualities of drummer/dancer interaction and the performance context. Out of respect for David and Noah's concern that I not give away details that would make it possible for outsiders to play Hong Luck's style, this transcription is more descriptive than prescriptive (Seeger 1958). Moreover, I have notated neither an extensive set of variations

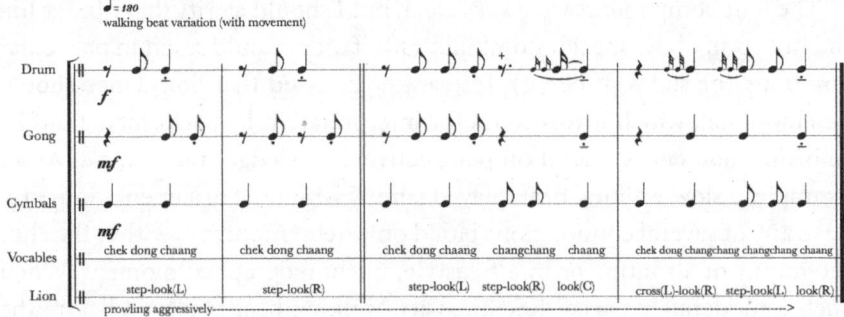

Figure 5.1 Inter-media walking-beat transcription with variation

Credits: Colin P. McGuire

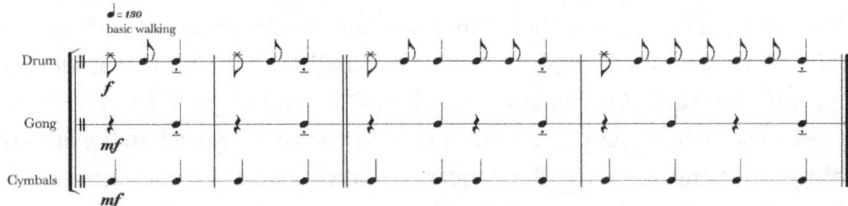

Figure 5.2 Basic walking-beat transcription

Credits: Colin P. McGuire

on one beat, nor a whole routine. As with the other transcriptions in this book, the notation does not represent a specific performance, but rather it showcases rhythms that have become part of my repertoire (i.e., they are transcribed from memory). For comparison, I have also transcribed a very basic walking pattern that more closely resembles the vocables (Figure 5.2).

In order to provide a rich transcription that reflects the four-part scheme, I include all three instruments, the vocables, and the lion's movement, but I remind the reader that vocables are not externalized in performance. My use of words to denote movement is adapted from Hai-Hsing Yao's (1990) work on percussion music for martial acrobatics in Chinese opera. The movement description focuses on where the lion is stepping and looking. In order to fit it into the notation I have abbreviated the directions as: L for left, R for right, and C for centre. The double bar line divides the transcription into two parts, with the second being twice as long as the first because, as previously discussed in Chapter 3, segmentation is based on drum/dance phrases and not on metre.

These transcriptions illustrate three main things. First is the relationship among the instruments. The cymbal part is the least demanding; it anchors the pulse with an even stream of quarter notes. While simple, it can still be challenging for some practitioners to maintain the pulse when there is as much variation as I have shown in the rich transcription, and this is why Master Jim encouraged David to moderate his drumming accordingly. The gong and drum parts allow more freedom than the cymbal parts do, but they are also responsible for indicating the vocable-driven structures and emphasizing the last beat of each phrase. The drummer must be particularly clear with this emphasis because the other percussionists follow the drummer's phrasing. I would also like to draw attention to the vocables in Figure 5.1, which resemble a composite of the three instrumental parts. This oral gong and drum text is closest to the basic walking beat learned by beginner lion dancers, which is like the drum part in Figure 5.2.

The second point to make about this transcription is that variations remain connected to the skeleton of the vocables. The gong line in Figure 5.1 shows offbeat syncopation in the second bar, something advanced performers might do to add rhythmic interest, particularly when not accompanying set choreography. In bars three and four of Figure 5.1, the drum line gives an example of variations created by mutes and rolls. The cross "+" sign above the quarter rest indicates a mute played as part of the rhythm (like Master Jim's chit), which is substituted for the beat that occurs there in the more basic version. Similarly, the rim clicks shown by an "x" in the basic transcription are omitted in the rich transcription, which is quite common in performance practice. The end of the third bar has what some drummers call an *under-roll*, or grace notes on the last beat, while the start of the fourth bar has what are sometimes referred to as *over-rolls*, or grace notes added to the first beat. These ornaments help to link bars three and four together into a combined phrase.

The third and final aspect to which I would like to draw attention is the phrasing of the lion dance steps and movements. Like the drum part, they are goal-oriented towards the end of phrases, but they do not always follow the drum rhythms exactly. For a simple, heartbeat-like drum pattern (i.e., the eighth rest, eighth note, and quarter note in the first two bars of Figure 5.1), lion footwork can mimic the drum by lifting the foot on the upbeat and landing on the downbeat. The drumming in bars three and four is more elaborate. The lion dance therefore does not—and often cannot—follow the drum patterns note for note, particularly when the drummer is selecting variants on the fly and further improvising variations with ornaments and/ or mutes. Instead, dancers draw on the drummer's intrinsic timing, style, and feeling, but their movement is often closer to the unspoken vocable pattern.

Training to Embody Martial Sound

In Chapter 4 I described how beginner kung fu students develop basic syn-chronization skills; I will now revisit this through a martial entrainment schema by connecting it to fighting applications. As in many martial arts, when Hong Luck novices drill basic strikes, blocks, and footwork, their teacher counts out loud and the pupils entrain their movement to the vocal stimulus. Synchronization is important here, and students are admonished if they end up ahead or behind the pulse set by the leader. This basic ability to entrain movement to an external source is as important for self-defence as it is for those who go on to lion dance training. Partner drills are limited in beginner's class, in part because they can be dangerous when students are still developing the ability to entrain. In cooperative attack-and-defence practice, each strike must be met with a homo-rhythmic block or evasion, which is also characteristic of applying successful defence skills in a real-life situation. Spatial and rhythmic synchronization thus undergirds students' success in partner drills where there is a risk of being struck. Through basic training in kung fu, the entrainment schema becomes a cognitive metaphor for how to protect oneself from physical violence, allowing practitioners to take stances on the meaning of (a)synchronicity.

Beginner class also features groupings of techniques into short combinations and, eventually, into longer choreographed forms. In ei-ther case, teachers initially count each movement individually, which effi-ciently organizes the use of space for training groups of people and continues to build entrainment skills. Once students become more familiar with the movements, however, instructors use only one verbal count per combination of basics or short section of a choreographed form. At that point, trainees start together, are no longer expected to stay in sync within a combina-tion, and then restart in time with one another on the teacher's next count. Depending on peoples' abilities and interpretations of the movement, there can be a high degree of asynchronicity inside the larger entrainment struc-ture. For basic training, the cycle of order and chaos is quite regular because each set of techniques is drilled repeatedly; the teacher's counting determines the points where students entrain with one another, and even though they naturally tend to become rhythmically independent inside combinations, the time interval is fairly steady for regrouping on the next count. That is to say, basic training tends to establish a pulse but allows asynchronicity within the subdivisions of each beat. This situation becomes increasingly complex in choreographed forms because each section of movement is different from the next and they are therefore of unequal length. The resulting constant-yet-erratic cycling between synchronicity and asynchronicity is character-istic of a martial entrainment schema, which becomes especially apparent for students who are allowed to join Hong Luck's sparring class.

As with lion dance, a solid foundation in traditional kung fu basics is the prerequisite for joining the sparring class. The coach for that session throughout my fieldwork was Adrian Balcă. As previously mentioned, Adrian won a gold medal in Canadian national sanshou competition, but he also has a wealth of experience acquired from self-defence situations on the street. He migrated from Romania as a young boy and was bullied by his classmates for being a foreigner with poor English skills. Adrian was no pushover, however, and he fought back, which is part of the reason he joined Hong Luck: he was looking to improve his fighting abilities. Master Paul Chan recognized the all-too-familiar pattern of discrimination and took this new Canadian under his wing. He coached Adrian in fighting applications, adding skill to the youngster's already pugnacious disposition. Hong Luck's sparring coach preserves the legacy of Hong Luck's tough history in Canada, guiding students through practical applications of martial arts rather than stance training or performing choreographed forms. Nonetheless, Adrian is strict about ensuring that new trainees have proved themselves in beginner class and have the approval of a teacher familiar with their abilities.

Notwithstanding the name, the "sparring" classes I attended rarely in-volved much free-fighting. Instead, they usually featured a self-directed warm-up and some shadowboxing drills as a group, before proceeding to structured applications of striking, grappling, and defence. We hit hand-held focus pads for accuracy, pounded on the heavy sandbags for power, and drilled semi-cooperative partner exercises for technique. Much less frequently, we donned protective gear and engaged in light-contact free-sparring.[2] Had my classmates and I been interested in entering kickboxing

---

[2] Senior members tell me that sparring at Hong Luck used to be much more regular and intense "back in the day," which appears to mean the 1980s to early 2000s. In the club's first two decades (1960s and 1970s), however, modern sanshou/sanda kickboxing was apparently less common than it was during my fieldwork.

competitions, Adrian would have been happy to tailor our training for that by having us spar more frequently. Nonetheless, bruises, scrapes, and strains were more common in sparring class than the rest of Hong Luck's curriculum, because every session involved contact with resisting partners and training equipment. Adrian also provided opportunities to explore applications of the techniques we were learning in Hong Luck's choreographed forms. I took advantage of these opportunities to investigate the rhythm of combat, which later opened up important avenues for thinking about martial sound in kung fu demonstrations.

Compared to the consistent entrainment of beginner class, the timing of the group members during sparring training was largely independent. Adrian assigned the techniques that we would work on, but he did not usually count them out. For basic techniques, shadowboxing, and bag-work, he merely set a number of repetitions or amount of time for practice but let us train at our own pace. This rhythmic freedom continued the progression from beginner class, where students were gradually given more opportunities for asynchronicity as they became familiar with the combinations. The gradual shift of entrainment during practice from synchronized to free can found in other martial arts as well. For example, John Donohue (2000) has remarked that within a Japanese kendo class, the audible contact of bamboo swords, sound of moving feet, and lusty yells are initially in sync during basic technique training; become more disordered during partner drills; and move towards sonic—and martial—chaos in the freestyle practice at the end of a session.

Adrian tended let us show him our stuff before offering feedback, although he was more amenable to answering questions than some of the more senior instructors. By mid-2013 I had been in his class for a few months, and I had become accustomed to modifying Hong Luck's kung fu basics according to the needs of practical application. At first, Adrian had me pursuing a greater economy of motion, by cutting out the exaggerated movements endemic to choreographed forms, adjusting my stances to cover distance flexibly, and striking powerfully without leaving myself vulnerable. As with most learners, I was drilling combinations of strikes like a metronomic automaton: one, two, three, pause, and repeat. Simple rhythms and repetition facilitate focusing one's attention on physical technique but are not ideal for combat. Eventually, Adrian began to coach me on the subtler aspects of hand combat.

My first challenge was to mix up striking patterns while training. Adrian explained that using the same attacking combinations over and over quickly becomes easy for an opponent to predict. Instead of compensating with a proliferation of different techniques, Adrian advocated working with a more limited palette of attacks but playing with their timing. To put his comment in perspective, Hong Luck's kung fu has a vast arsenal of techniques, but we only focused on the most practical ones in sparring class, leaving the more esoteric methods for choreographed forms. Nonetheless, the range of skills covered in Adrian's class far exceeded what could legally be used in any type of kickboxing competition. To make his point about rhythmic variation of striking combinations clearer, he then used vocables to speak some examples. These were not oral gong and drum texts, but rather onomatopoeic approximations of punches and kicks landing. Over the next several months, Adrian sometimes asked me to express in words the timing methods he demonstrated in class, recognizing that musical terms might prove helpful for explaining the rhythm of combat. He also expressed an interest in hearing what sort of rhythmic possibilities I might work out for myself.

Hearing the Rhythm of Combat

From Hong Luck's training floor to the coaching that happens between rounds in MMA, rhythm is frequently mentioned in combative practices, but rarely explained in detail. Two historical examples are rare exceptions to this lacuna. Just before his death in 1645, an undefeated Japanese samurai named Miyamoto Musashi wrote a series of letters to his student; these were later compiled as *The Book of Five Rings*. This text contains both theoretical and practical advice on the warrior's path, including several references to the importance of rhythm. Musashi wrote, "[v]ictory is achieved in the *Heihō* of conflict by ascertaining the rhythm of each opponent, by attacking with a rhythm not anticipated by the opponent, and by use of knowledge of the rhythm of the abstract" (1982: 25).[3] Musashi even made explicit reference to rhythm in music and dance as models for understanding timing in martial arts. He also wrote, "[f]rom one thing, know ten thousand things" (1982: 21), which is not unlike the idea of a durable habitus built from the economical transferability of practical logic. More recently, the work of martial artist and

---

[3] The Japanese word *heihō* [兵法] literally means *military methods* but is more accurately translated as the *art of war*. Musashi uses it to refer to the warrior's path, which he sees as a road to achieving enlightenment.

movie star Bruce Lee has presented a sustained practical engagement with the topic of rhythm in combat (Lee 1975: 59–67). His approach to martial arts was eclectic and syncretic, which is reflected in his writing on timing. Lee appears to have drawn his terminology from a combination of military drill, music, fencing, and chess, which unfortunately makes his exposition inconsistent in some places. I have engaged with Lee's work in more detail elsewhere (McGuire 2019), so I will leave that discussion aside for now.

Poststructuralists tend to see all human experience as text, but some modes of expression are better suited to being heard as music, such as hand combat. Simon Frith has criticized reading events as text in favour of close attention to context, and further suggested that postmodernists "have more to learn from a study of popular music than popular music theorists have to learn from postmodernism" (1996: 204). My concept of martial sound presents a way of discussing the experience of physical culture as music and a means of listening to the context of combative events. Moreover, thinking musically about martial arts has been of great interest to my consultants, as compared to the reticence some of them have shown towards discussing the tong system or documenting their gong and drum repertoire with music notation.

Building on my previous work (McGuire 2010), I propose that musical vocabulary offers a readymade, self-consistent, precise way of talking about the rhythm of combat, which is central to my concept of martial sound. Timing is how one knows when to act in order to achieve one's aims, and it is at the core of martial being-in-time. Strategic control of timing is essential in martial arts of all varieties, whether in combat sports where timing determines the outcome of a competition, or in choreographed forms where timing shapes the success of a performance. As previously mentioned, successful defence relies on being able to entrain one's movement to that of the opponent, whether through evasions, deflections, blocks, traps, stuffs, or sprawls. As a strike or takedown attempt comes in, a defence must be synchronized with the attack in order to escape, parry, absorb, or control it. Seen from the opposite angle, successful attacks must use a variety of rhythms and a flexible tempo to circumvent an opponent's defences. Avoiding entrainment is thus central to the timing of offensive footwork, punches, kicks, knees, elbows, pokes, pushes, grabs, traps, locks, trips, throws, takedowns, and so on. Martial sound allows us to hear sonic and kinetic timing, which opens it up to musical analysis that reveals the rhythms of combat, choreomusical connections, and entrainment relationships.

Under Adrian's guidance, I explored a staple Choi Lee Fut punching combination as a case study on how we can hear combat musically through martial sound, the results of which are mapped in Figure 5.3. The combination is comprised of three strikes: a lead backfist or "hanging punch" [*gwaa chèuih*, 掛捶], a rear cross or "piercing punch" [*chyūn chèuih*, 穿捶], and a lead overhand or "sweeping punch" [*sau chèuih*, 捎捶]. The English names of these punches come from kickboxing, where *lead* refers to the side of a fighter's body that is closest to the opponent/target and *rear* is the side farther away. To map striking combinations with music notation requires determining the basic unit of pulse, which in hand combat is the duration of a simple movement, such as taking a step, launching a punch, or punching while stepping (Lee 1975:60–61). Tempo tends to fluctuate in fighting much more than it does in most types of music because combatants are constantly vying to control timing. Within a single combination, however, the rate of pulse stabilizes somewhat, if only momentarily. In Figure 5.3, I present a non-exhaustive range of rhythmic options for this three-punch combination. The notes above the line are for the lead hand and those below are for the rear hand. The single line staffs reflect the percussive nature of striking. Each note expresses an intended point of impact—whether successfully landed or not.

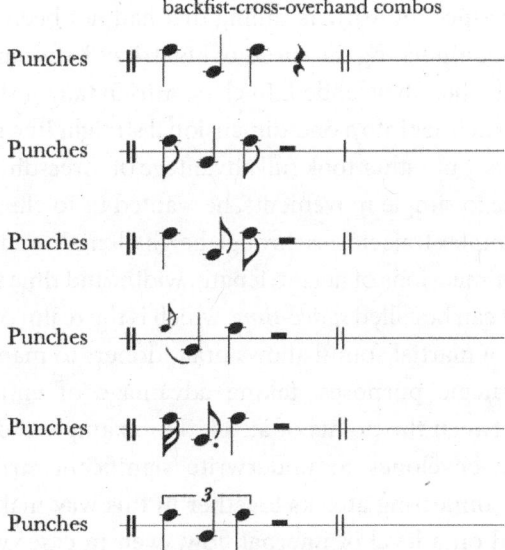

Figure 5.3 Transcription of punching combination rhythms
Credits: Colin P. McGuire

For the sake of simplicity, this brief analysis focuses only on striking and does not take stepping, feinting, or defending into account. A quarter note is given as the basic pulse of movement-time, and I avoid micro-subdivisions to focus on the most archetypal rhythms.

In discussing the possibility of a common vocabulary for music and dance, Jörgen Torp (2013) has emphasized the need to consider what happens between events. Conveniently for my purposes, he uses the word *attack* when referring to both the beginning of a sound and the arrival of a movement. It may be convenient to think of a rhythm (sonic or kinetic) as a series of attacks that make a pattern in time, but Torp points out that these points are inconceivable without the connections between them. It is in those connections that we find the "movement character of flowing rhythm" (Torp 2013: 240), which is as important as the pattern of attacks. In hand combat, the space-time trajectory of an attack belies a seemingly simple rhythm pattern.

At the last sparring class before Christmas break in 2013, Adrian let me video record him punching, kicking, elbowing, and pushing the heavy bag, which helped to reveal how the flow of movement over time connects points of a combative rhythm in non-linear ways. Just as Western music notation does not capture the timbral complexities within an individual note, it could conceal the flowing intricacies of an individual strike, so it is important to listen between the attacks. After watching the video clip several times, I eventually noticed a subtle aspect of Adrian's timing that had not been apparent to me before. He was manipulating the speed of his strikes between their initiation and the moment when they landed. In class, Adrian taught striking methods that were locked neither into a one-dimensional straight line nor into a swing across two planes, but rather took full advantage of three-dimensional space. While not averse to simple movements, he wanted us to alternate them with attacks along complex trajectories through height, length, and width. By combining the four dimensions of height, length, width, and time into one parameter, we get what can be called *space-time*, which is the realm of martial sound.

A firm grasp of martial sound allows practitioners to manipulate flowing rhythm for strategic purposes, taking advantage of entrainment while subverting it between the points of attack. For example, Adrian uses complex space-time envelopes to underwrite significant strikes within his combinations. Connecting attacks together in this way makes them rhythmically nuanced on a level of internal flow, even in cases where the more obvious points of impact create a basic rhythmic pattern. In light sparring with Adrian, I experienced his control of martial sound as a constant misjudgment of where my defence should be. In essence, his complex space-time envelopes allowed him to move slightly out of phase with, or to syncopate against, a pattern of his own creation, which thwarted my attempts to entrain blocks or evasions. His manipulations of rhythmic flow could swerve to land just ahead of my parry and could dawdle long enough to enter on an opening that my defence created.

Not everyone at Hong Luck is as musical in their martial arts as Adrian. At the fifty-third anniversary, one senior member told me he used to play the drum but had to stop because, "it was messing up my punching." He argued that the relatively constant tempo and repetitive nature of Hong Luck's percussion rhythms were not conducive to fighting, which is true in one sense, but not in another. The rhythm of combat is not exactly the same as in music; being rhythmically unpredictable is often desirable in a fight, but detrimental to a musical ensemble. Nonetheless, establishing predictable combat rhythm patterns or keeping a steady pace of fighting moves can be used to bait an opponent into a vulnerable position by leading their movement to entrainment. This senior member's cognitive separation of music and kung fu suggests that not everyone is willing—or able—to draw on the commonalities between them.

Similarly, one of Adrian's sparring partners is terrible at playing lion dance percussion, but he is still an excellent fighter. He is a senior at Hong Luck and now runs his own club, so I was quite surprised when I heard him play cymbals one day. I observed that his timing was weak, and consistent entrainment to the beat of the drum appeared to elude him. When I had the chance to see him spar, however, I observed how he used that apparent rhythmic deficit to his advantage by shutting down his opponent's ability to entrain. He charged forward and immediately contacted his opponent, and then stifled him with an unsteady stream of arrhythmic grabs, pushes, and strikes. I have not sparred with him myself, but this senior member is apparently quite difficult to defend against because of the smothering pressure and violent lack of regularity. I bring up the last two examples in order to show that martial sound need not be musical to be effective.

Martial Sound in Embodied Strategy

Hand combat is unpredictable; it happens too fast for fighters to methodically count, analyze, and regulate rhythm, which is why martial sound strategies must become embodied responses before they can be applied. Through assiduous training, patterns of movement and timing become so engrained that fighters can use them instinctively (Spencer 2009; Wacquant 2004). In the practice hall, strategy must guide the development of technique so that it can be used tactically in combat. Participants in combat sports and unwilling victims of physical assault defending themselves are both more likely to be successful if their training has guided them to an embodied understanding of how to set up an attack and how to proactively defend, rather than prioritizing mechanical perfection of technique (Kozub and Kozub 2004). This premise is logical if one considers that a mechanically flawed attack launched at the right time is more likely to score than a technically perfect attack initiated when there is no opening.

When I asked Adrian about his uncanny timing, his explanation revealed the strategic implications of a Chinese way-of-being martial in time. He explained that a combination of three-dimensional movement with control of speed allows him to change course and/or velocity at any time until the final impact. At the last possible movement, he could then add power by shifting his stance and body weight, which would condense space-time in an explosive acceleration. Adrian used the term *fajing* to explain the method, which is Mandarin for "emit power" [*faat gihng*, 發勁]. This type of movement belongs to what I described in the Chapter 4 as the calligraphy-like flow that Master Paul Chan had scolded me about when he said my kung fu needed to be more Chinese. Another way of thinking about this embodied strategy would be as rhythmic counterpoint. Advanced practitioners are able to hear their opponent's combative rhythms through martial sound, which allows them to anticipate entrained defences and improvise a counterrhythm. Doing so requires the ability to connect points of attack with flowing rhythm in order to expand space-time before compressing it into a devastating blow.

In the video of Adrian hitting the heavy-bag, I noticed that he was also using abrupt tempo shifts where he would throw a few combinations at one steady pace and then suddenly follow up at different speed. I know from class that Hong Luck's sparring coach does not advocate the use of false attacks to establish a tempo or draw reactions from the opponent. Instead, he recommends always using real attacks because they get a stronger reaction, and, even when thrown with fifty percent power, they can cause damage. Adrian's strategy contrasts with Bruce Lee's recommendation to use feinting as a means to establish a tempo (1975: 64). Despite the contrast of stances on how best to dictate the pace of a fight, the goal of both methods is to entrain the opponent's tempo. Watching the video of Adrian hitting the heavy-bag, I could see how he might lull an opponent into a false sense of security with a steady, predictable pace of half-strength attacks and then flatten them with unexpectedly powerful techniques at a different tempo. Interestingly, he did not always speed up for the decisive strike. In some cases, he slowed down, which would still have the effect of catching an opponent vulnerable while they momentarily remained entrained to a different tempo.[4]

Pace of movement-time can be a weapon—even when it is steady. The tempo of hand combat is often highly unstable, because it fluctuates both while opponents vie for positional advantage and during moments of engagement, as well as according to the ebb and flow of their energy levels. In some cases, it would be difficult to identify a pulse of movement-time at all. At other times, however, tempo can be rock-steady for strategic purposes. An example was recounted to me in the summer of 2014 by a student from a martial arts school founded by a Hong Luck alumnus. This student still practised traditional kung fu, but he was more focused on competing in sanda/sanshou kickboxing. He suggested that his natural quickness usually gave him a speed advantage over his opponents, and he combined this with his excellent physical conditioning and reserve of stamina to use tempo tactically. He would push the pace of a match, steadily outworking his opponents with a barrage of feints and strikes until they became tired. Then, he would take his tempo up a notch and overwhelm them with strikes to win the fight.

Another way that Adrian taught strategic concepts with martial sound was when highlighting the need for diversity in striking. For example, he sometimes talked about striking combinations as a melody that needs different notes. Lacking the musical vocabulary to explain a combative melody in greater depth, Adrian has had more success using Hong Luck's percussion as a metaphor instead. He suggested that, in addition to rhythm, both a percussion ensemble and a fighting combination need to have a variety of "tones," whether to create interesting motifs or devastating attacks. He talked about the drum being low pitched, while the gong is medium high, and the cymbals are high, which he mapped onto the targets of an opponent's body being low, middle, or high. When applying strikes to various targets, the

---

[4] A reduction of tempo in the final strike could potentially reduce its power, but it would still be effective against an opponent who is moving forwards because the velocity of the strike would be amplified by the adversary's incoming movement.

strategy is to get into tonal counterpoint with the opponent's defence while entraining rhythmic unison. The first successful strike establishes the basis for a tonal pattern that is maintained even while being subverted. When an attack causes pain, the instinctive reaction is to defend that line, which opens up the next target because no one can defend their whole body at once. Each successive attack is then entrained with the defence, but lands at a different location than the spot being defended. Sensible in theory, the efficacy of this martial sound strategy was abundantly clear when our teacher did it to me. In sparring, Adrian's assault beat me as though my whole body was a set of percussion: head, torso, arms, and legs. Sure enough, as soon as he struck me and I moved to defend the place where I had been hurt, he would hit me somewhere else. Furthermore, his barrage was delivered in a variety of attacking rhythms, using both simple and complex space-time envelopes. Even with light contact, the way he could impose his timing was terrifying, and it felt like my own efforts at defence were being used against me.

Master Jim was already in his eighties when I had the privilege of training with him,[5] and what he lacked in physicality was covered by strategy and his deep well of experience. In demonstrating technique to us, he could still use position and timing tactically to compensate for a lack of speed or power. In particular, he deployed two strategies that are common among various styles of kung fu: "linking defence to attack" [lìhn sīu daai dá, 連消帶打], meaning to use defence as attack or attack as defence; and "move first gain initiative" [sīn faat jai yàhn, 先發制人], which means to act before one's opponent(s) in order to control timing, whether by catching them off-guard, by feinting to get a reaction, or by beating them to the punch. Master Jim was not one to use four-character "set idioms" [sìhngyúh, 成語] with students, perhaps because of language barriers between English, Cantonese, and his native Taishanese, but these sayings nonetheless match the meaning of his explanations and demonstrations. The entrainment schema impinges directly on these two strategies, and I can use martial sound to help explain them.

Within Master Jim's choreographed Choi Lee Fut kung fu hand forms, any technique that is repeated three times in a row will have a distinctive rhythm pattern, which has strategic implications. The time distance between the

---

[5] Hong Luck members who trained with Master Jim in his physical prime told me stories about his exploits. Apparently, his iron-like arms allowed him to turn the tide of a fight without throwing a punch because his defensive manoeuvres were themselves crushing blows. I also heard how he once used the movement pattern from his signature Cross-Shaped Boxing [Sahp Jih Kyùhn, 十字拳] form to fight off multiple attackers during an altercation.

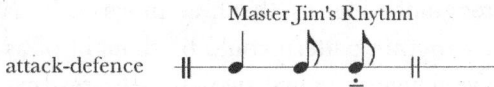

Figure 5.4 Master Jim's rhythm
Credits: Colin P. McGuire

first two moves is double the duration between the second and third (musically: quarter–eighth–eighth), and some senior members have even clapped it out for me (see the transcription in Figure 5.4). Master Jim demonstrated this pattern with a strong accent on the last move and a slight acceleration to the finish. As a combative rhythm, the first two notes establish a tempo, as well as the expectation that the next note will follow the same pattern of landing right on a beat. The third move breaks the pattern, however, by arriving on an offbeat. We need only think of a conductor giving just an upbeat and a downbeat to establish tempo for an orchestra to see how little rhythmic information people actually need to entrain a pulse.[6] The strategy works by foiling an opponent's expectation that the time between move two and three will be the same as between one and two. Essentially, Master Jim's three-beat rhythm embodies Bruce Lee's most famous timing strategy, which he dubbed *broken rhythm* (1975). To reiterate, in a combative stalemate, each attack is met with a homo-rhythmic defence, and so neither opponent can gain the upper hand. Using a broken rhythm means to strike outside of a pattern of entrainment, while the opponent continues with it just long enough to get caught. Control of timing through broken rhythm strategy goes a long way to overcoming a deficit of physical speed.

Master Jim's rhythm can be applied in attack or defence, and it allows one to move first in order to gain initiative in altercation. For example, the "eagle claw" [*yīngjáu*, 鷹爪] was his favoured open-hand technique, and it came up as a thrice-repeated move in several of his choreographed forms. Physically, it uses the thumb, index, and middle fingers to form a "claw" and can be either an attack or a defence. In blocking, one partially extends the arm to contact an opponent's strike, which is usually combined with footwork called "triangle stepping" [*sāamgok máah*, 三角馬] to deflect an attacker's force at

6 I must give credit to Dr. Jessica Cawley for providing the example of how quickly and efficiently conductors can establish a tempo. She was also careful to point out that less professional ensembles might still require a full bar count-in to prepare them.

an angle. In choreographed forms, the three-move eagle claw combinations using Master Jim's rhythm pattern could be thought of as two deflections followed by an eye-gouge. The first two are defences that create a homo-rhythmic stalemate while the third is a counterattack that breaks the pattern. Master Jim was at pains to emphasize to us that one should never block attacks more than twice without mounting a counteroffensive. Rather than suggesting continuous defence, I hear the rhythm as representing a strategy of finding the opponent's tempo and rhythm pattern, then acting first before they can make their next move in order to seize the initiative.

Notwithstanding the presence of this three-beat pattern in choreographed forms, Master Jim distilled the strategy as a single beat for free-fighting applications. When he showed us how to apply his eagle claw for self-defence, he said to avoid wasting time on blocking by linking defence to attack. His demonstrations used one continuous motion that blocked the attack and, using the same hand, continued with a counterattack—without resetting or withdrawing. In order for this to work, one must intercept an incoming strike halfway through its motion and follow up before the opponent is able to make a second move. Both the defence and counterstroke are syncopated sharply against the adversary's attack as a broken rhythm. Although technically the opponent initiated, the idea is to interrupt their movement and finish before they do, thus seizing the initiative. Bruce Lee refers to this strategy as a *stop-hit*, "a timed hit made against the adversary at the same time he is making an attack. It *anticipates and intercepts* the final line of attack" (italics in original, 1975: 65). The strategy works particularly well against attackers who use a lot of feints because one can stop-hit with impunity against a fake attack, but it also works nicely against heavy hitters who are powerful but slow.

In this chapter, I have discussed how Hong Luck members experience martial sound through embodied understandings of kung fu and lion dance. Specifically, I introduced and applied the entrainment schema as a cognitive metaphor, as well as explained Master Jim's four-part division of lion dance's choreomusical meaning. In delving deeper into martial entrainment, I have explored how training inculcates embodied knowledge of combative rhythms. I have also analyzed some of the key strategies that allow martial sound to be applied tactically in hand combat. In the next chapter, I bring my own participant perspective to the interpretation of martial sound in kung fu demos, lion dance, and drumming, extending embodied knowledge of entrainment to interpret the realm of performance.

6

Experiencing Martial Sound
in Performance

The Horizons of Awareness

Peak performance experiences provide exceptionally rich ethnographic examples of martial sound. At Hong Luck, the highlight of the club's annual calendar is its anniversary celebration in August, which is a full-day event that includes a lion dance parade through Chinatown, as well as a ten-course banquet with martial arts demonstrations and even more lion dance performances. The kung fu demonstrations involve choreographed forms accompanied by percussion, which is a relative rarity; for many members, it is the only time of the year (apart from dress rehearsals just before the anniversary) that they ever do martial arts with percussion accompaniment or perform in public. This situation presents some special challenges that I describe, explain, and interpret according to entrainment metaphors of (a) synchronicity vis-à-vis the rhythm of combat. I also discuss the main lion dance performance at the banquet, with special attention to the entrainment schema and Master Jim's four elements. Finally, I examine the experience of drumming, which I extend beyond the bounds of the anniversary. This chapter follows the expanding awareness of situation and entrainment for the performer in each of these three areas (kung fu, lion dance, and drumming), starting with the narrowest perceptual horizon during martial arts demonstrations.

The three case studies in this chapter are phenomenological descriptions of my experiences performing Hong Luck's blurred genre. These ethnographic vignettes are more extensive than elsewhere in the book, and, while I use a phenomenological attitude to reveal these practices as given in experience, they are not a purely subjective interpretation. I maintain that the elders and seniors at Hong Luck have shaped my corporeal understanding through the apprenticeship process, thus rendering the descriptions intersubjective.

Martial Sound. Colin P. McGuire, Oxford University Press. © Oxford University Press 2024.
DOI: 10.1093/oso/9780197775936.003.0006

(A)synchronicity in Martial Arts Demos

I was quite nervous the first time I performed kung fu at a Hong Luck anniversary, which was in 2010, around two years after I joined the club. Despite near daily solo practice during the six weeks leading up to the banquet, performing kung fu with drum accompaniment turned out to be more of a challenge than one might expect. In class, I had earned my teacher's confidence with an empty-hand Choi Lee Fut form called Small Plum-Flower Boxing [*Síu Mùihfā Kyùhn*, 小梅花拳] and was assigned to perform it at the anniversary banquet. During dress rehearsals in the two weeks before the big day, however, I was overwhelmed when trying to perform kung fu while the gong and drum ensemble pummeled me with martial sound. Every time I got up in front of my classmates to do my demonstration, I struggled to remember choreography that I could do in silence without difficulty.

After I forgot the moves halfway through on back-to-back attempts, my teacher from the beginner class, Quang, gave me two important pieces of advice. First, he showed me how to bow out if I forgot my form while performing on stage, suggesting that I try to make it look like that was actually the end of the form so that non-practitioners in the audience might not know the difference. Second, he told me that the trick to performing with the percussion ensemble is not to follow the drum. Quang explained that I needed to maintain my own kung fu rhythm because the fast, powerful beats are intended to provide motivation, not guide movement. The rhythms are essentially variants on lion dance beats (walking and head-up) that emphasize intrinsic martial qualities: power, speed, volume, and aggression. Although drummers may play somewhat more gently and simply when accompanying younger and/or less experienced performers, the stylistic requirements for kung fu drumming typically call for some sonic intensity. Quang's advice highlighted a distinctive choreomusical relationship, namely for sound and movement to remain largely asynchronous (with a few key exceptions) while still sharing the same energy. Over the next several years, numerous Hong Luck seniors echoed his message about the importance of a performer's combative rhythms remaining independent from the gong and drum ensemble.

I will engage with meanings that arise from the concept of choreomusical asynchronicity after I describe the experience of a specific event. My performance at the 2010 anniversary was minimally acceptable, as evidenced by Master Paul's grudging "OK," and I eventually became more capable of giving kung fu demonstration on stage. Nonetheless, the drumming-fuelled adrenaline surge has continued to be as intense as ever, and choreomusical asynchronicity remains challenging. At Hong Luck's fifty-third anniversary in 2014, I performed one of Master Jim's more advanced choreographed forms called Dragon Boxing [*Lùhng Kyùhn*, 龍拳]:

The MC announces, "Colin McGuire performing Luhng Kyuhn." I take a deep breath, then leave my position with the instruments and other performers to make my way towards centre stage. Meanwhile, Noah softly beats out a special variation of the walking beat that's used to introduce kung fu demos. As I arrive at the middle of the stage, he dramatically gives three sharp rim-clicks to cue the beginning of my demo. I lift my hands in a Shaolin salute to the audience of the packed banquet hall, and my heart is pounding in my chest . . . I soften my awareness of the crowd, filled with my juniors, peers, and teachers, as well as various kung fu masters, local dignitaries, and guests. Now they're just a fuzzy, undifferentiated mass, and I hear Noah begin a continuous drum roll. On cue, I reel my fists back through the air and chamber them at my waist. I look down briefly to compose myself before launching into the opening bows of Master Jim's Dragon Boxing form. Step-by-step, I carefully proceed at a measured pace; the intro is a time for clarity and poise. I finish the opening by rolling my fists to my waist a second time, which I entrain to a three-beat rhythmic cadence from Noah: *chek-dong-chit*.

Suddenly, fast and furious martial sound explodes from the percussionists. I feel a potent rush of power shoot up my spine that momentarily threatens to overwhelm me . . . my mind goes blank . . . then suddenly my awareness further narrows to tunnel vision as I compress all that energy down into my centre. Embodied memory takes over, my face twists into a snarl, and I explode into a flurry of combat moves. I no longer hear the drumming as specific rhythms, but rather feel it as an insistent, pulsing wave of sound pushing me forwards. I punch, kick, jump, spin, and coil, punctuating the ends of combinations with ferocious yells. The imaginary opponents receiving this onslaught are shredded by my eagle claws and smashed by my strikes.

Un-distracted by the beats, I assert my own combative rhythm, which flirts with entrainment to the drum at several points, only to swerve out of phase again. Noah pushes me relentlessly onwards with his drumming, sometimes changing his variations to emphasize my combinations, and we drive hard towards the end of the form. At the penultimate combination, I'm facing the back of the stage where two Hong Luck banners are draped under the restaurant's dragon and phoenix wall decorations. I don't even see them. Finally, I lunge into a 180-degree hook punch that turns me back towards the audience for a finishing blow. I violently unleash it with a feral bellow that erupts from deep within me and my fifty-five seconds of kung fu are done. The furor of performance dissipates, and I can see more than a few raised eyebrows in the audience. As I roll my fists back to my waist for the third and final time, Noah repeats the rhythmic cadence and we end in sync: *chek-dong-chit*. I give one more Shaolin bow and exit the stage to the sound of applause.

To interpret the choreomusical meanings of martial sound in kung fu performances, I return to the embodied knowledge transmitted through Hong Luck's training program. In sparring class, I saw how remaining asynchronous or in counterpoint to an opponent's defence is integral to landing successful attacks. When I asked Adrian, the sparring coach, whether martial arts demonstrations with percussion accompaniment could benefit a practitioner's combative timing, he did not hesitate to confirm that it would. In his view, all aspects of kung fu as a blurred genre are martial arts, although some are more practical than others. Adrian suggested that being self-reflexive is the key to identifying transferable aspects and interconnections among Hong Luck's diverse range of practices.

The martial entrainment schema provides a central cognitive metaphor to both hand combat and kung fu demos with percussion accompaniment. As a combatant or performer, one must be aware of the rhythms one confronts without succumbing to them, which I can attest is difficult whether in relation to a crafty opponent or powerful drumming. In either case, avoiding entrainment requires splitting one's perceptual focus into foreground and background. Effective attacks in hand combat and successful kung fu demonstrations alike rely on asynchronicity, but they also use a small degree of entrainment in order to avoid it on a larger scale. It is necessary to acknowledge the opposing rhythm in order to maintain independence from it, to be in the rhythm but not of the rhythm. Drummers, however, are not required to play their beats asynchronously to the movement of a demo, which makes the percussion rhythms into something of an opponent. Percussionists accompany and motivate kung fu performers while providing a martial mood or atmosphere for the performance. The onus is on the person doing the demonstration to manifest the rhythm of combat. An exception to the general goal of asynchronicity is the introductory and concluding bows of a choreographed form. In these sections, drummer and performer work together to put up a unified front by entraining to each other, as I described in the ethnographic vignette above.

In Hong Luck's kung fu, there is room for personal flair in choreographed forms, and thus there are exceptions to the general pattern of asynchronicity that I have described. Some senior members take a more theatrical approach that involves exaggerated movements such as higher kicks, bigger punches, open postures, and affected gestures. Important to that exaggeration is synchronization with the percussion on certain movements, which enhances the dramatic effect. Such theatrics can look nice, but they present kung fu in a way that is less practical for fighting. Master Jim was highly critical of "flowery punches and embroidery kicks" [*fā kyùhn sau téui*, 花拳繡腿], a derogatory name for martial arts that look good but are combatively useless. Instead, he wanted to see real power, efficient speed, and practical technique, reserving drama for fierce yells and piercing eyes. One long-time member, approved by Master Jim, favoured a slightly exaggerated style of demonstration. In the advanced class, he warned me that there are limits to how far one could—or should—go with personal flair. Echoing Master Jim, he said that kung fu must remain grounded in fighting application or else it would cease to be a martial art. In his view, a bit of synchronization to the beat looks good at points of emphasis like poses or on the end of combinations. At the same time, this senior member opined that too much synchronization with the percussion would turn kung fu into a dance and would therefore be wrong. This more nuanced view of timing and intention in kung fu demonstrations goes beyond the simple advice given to beginners (i.e., do not follow the drum). Nonetheless, over time I have observed many performances—from both novices and seniors alike—that lacked a combative feeling because the performers had fallen into entrainment with the percussions. While these were not necessarily total failures, the dance-like approach of following the beat remains antithetical to the ideal of Hong Luck's combat-oriented performance practice.

More rarely, some choreographed kung fu forms actually require dramatic synchronization. General Guan's Halberd [*Jēung Gwāan Daaih Dōu*, 將關大刀], for example, has sections where the drummer should change the beat to accent the movement. These dramatic episodes are interspersed within the choreographed fighting skills and include riding a "horse," surveying a "battlefield" while stroking a long "beard," and sharpening the halberd on the ground before plucking a "hair" from the performer's own head to test the edge. Skilled drummers like Frank Ng can help dramatize martial arts demonstrations by playing a rhythm that aligns with dramaturgical movement; and experienced kung fu performers try to synchronize their movement with the drumming in theatrical parts of a form. Although drummer and martial artist must cooperate in order entrain to each other, the leader is the person doing kung fu. This dramaturgical approach is reminiscent of the way percussionists accompany the martial acrobatic arts found in Chinese opera (Yao 1990, 2001), where the choreomusical relationship privileges movement and requires sound to follow. Despite brief moments of entrainment in Hong Luck's forms, I would like to re-emphasize that the general practice for kung fu demonstrations with percussion accompaniment centres on asynchronicity. On average, synchronizing only accounts for between 10 and 20 percent of a successful demonstration, depending on the form, the performer, and the drummer.

Lion Dance Soldiers

Lion dancing requires a more entrained relationship to the drum rhythms than is required in demonstrating kung fu forms. As is common in dance styles around the world, lion dance is synchronized with the beat. This is not to say that every movement must coincide exactly with the drum rhythms, but rather that the tempo, feel, direction, and sequence of the dance are determined by the drumming. The martial arts context of the training environment lends another meaning to lion dance entrainment—one that is beholden to the percussion ensemble's origins as instruments of war. A drummer is like the general of an army who gives signals to troops on an ancient battlefield. Soldiers mired in the havoc of a fray would have been blind to the bigger picture of a battle, and they would have relied on drum signals for orientation. Similarly, lion costumes cover dancers' eyes, preventing them from seeing what is around them. In lion dancing, martial sound not only cues choreography, but also provides crucial information to orient performers to their surroundings. The following description depicts my experience of martial sound while doing the main lion dance of the evening at Hong Luck's fifty-third anniversary banquet:

I'm on the stage waiting to start. It's an honour to be under one of the two lion heads for plucking-the-greens, but I'm almost ready to drop from exhaustion. Almost. I already did a five-hour lion dance parade in the afternoon and two kung fu demos earlier in the banquet, so I have to dig deep as I steel myself for one more performance.

Noah is going to do the other head, and we are standing next to each other with the lions on the ground to our respective right-hand sides. He gives a loud shout to bring the two tail-dancers and myself to attention. David starts playing a continuous roll while we do a very short kung fu bow before getting under the heads. I'm doubly honoured tonight because I'm using a special, black and red, Guan Yu lion that only comes out once a year for the anniversary. It's larger and more ornate than the ones we usually use, which also makes it heavier. Once I slip it over me, I ignore the added bulk and treat it like an extension of my own body.

As we start the routine, I try to sink into my usual horse stance—and fail. My hips seize up, shooting pain through my legs . . . I wince and grit my teeth but am forced to stand taller than I should. Maybe they'll loosen up . . . David continues rolling on the drum as he waits for cues from us in the first section of the dance, which is one of the few parts where the lions lead the instruments. From behind the mask, I can hardly see what's in front of me. I only catch glimpses through a couple of slits where the lion's eyeballs are attached to the bamboo frame and also through the opening for the mouth. Luckily, Noah and I can see each other's feet from under the head, which works in this section because we're side-by-side and not walking anywhere. We sync our movement from horse stance into a crane stance, finishing together on a dampened drum accent from David. This pattern is repeated two more times before we start following the drum. It's much easier to coordinate when we can just listen to the beat. Next David plays a long version of the lion bow rhythm and we do three steps forwards while rolling the heads in a broad circle ending at the floor, and then shuffle back to our starting position with the masks kept low to the ground. As we bow, I use smooth, measured movements that embody the extra respect this drum signal calls for.

With an explosive rimshot, David starts the dance proper and launches into a head-up rhythm. Again, I try to get down in my horse stance but fail. I'm still blocked with pain in my hips and uncooperative muscles. Luckily, we don't stay there for long as a three-rises rhythm comes to my rescue. Next comes a side-to-side shuffle, which David calls for with a straight stream of heavy quarter notes—suddenly, however, he pulls out an old-school varia-tion! I've heard it before, but never danced to it . . . just as I'm about to lose my place in the choreography, I can almost hear Master Jim's voice telling me to mind the lion dance's four elements. I suddenly become aware of the vocables. They've been there the whole time—somewhere between or be-hind the drumming and movement—and I switch my focus to latch onto them. When I get to the crossover step that needs to finish on exactly the right drumbeat, I'm pleased to find that everything lines up.

Sweat is dripping into my eyes, but at least my muscle cramps are subsiding now that I'm getting warmed up again. We finish the routine and David plays a quiet walking beat at a slightly slower tempo. I start looking around for the greens that I will pluck. With limited vision and the rule of staying under the lion head while performing, searching for food can be tricky. I can't find the greens at first, but finally spy the restaurant staff getting them ready, so I prowl about the stage a bit more and trust that David will cue us when the veggies arrive.

Finally, David starts playing louder again as a dignitary makes his way towards us with the lettuce dangling from a string tied to a stick. Instead of going directly after the food, however, Noah and I start a lion fight. Much to the crowd's delight, we kick, bite, and push each other for a bit until he backs down, as we'd planned before the performance. We're brother lions, but when there's food involved the aggression comes out and I'm a little overzealous with my final roundhouse kick: oops! I then cautiously ap-proach the greens, and David stops leading as I take control of the per-formance. This sequence is the highlight of the routine, so I take my time. David accompanies me with continuous rolls that he modulates with volume swells to match the energy of my movements. When I make sig-nificant moves like sniffing the food or suddenly retreating, David marks them with accent strokes on the drum before returning to his rolling. I take a snap at the food, sniff the VIP, and finally do my signature double jump front-kick towards the lettuce before deciding it's safe to eat.

After plucking the greens, I catch my breath as I prepare to "chew," "swallow," "spit," and do the grand finale. Quickly, I remove the red packet and put it in between my teeth for safekeeping. Then, I tear the veggies into pieces and press them against the lion head's lower jaw with the mouth of the mask closed. When I tilt the head back to let David know I'm ready, we switch our choreomusical relationship again, and I start following him on the swallowing and spitting beats. At the end of the sequence, I open the lion mouth and catapult lettuce pieces onto the table in front of centre stage. David then cues the finale with extra fast, loud, head-up beats. I'm a happy lion after eating. I not only shake the head vigorously in the air, but also sink into my deepest stance, shifting my weight back and forth to put extra motion into the mask. What little energy I had left is already spent; there is nothing keeping me going but drumbeats, honour, and willpower. Nonetheless, I somehow finish strong, do three bows, and it's over. Now that the lion has eaten, it's time for the dancers to feast, too!

As the preceding description shows, lion dancers' situational awareness is spatial and aural because their visual field is limited. They cannot rely on vision while under the head, and thus hearing becomes more important. Dancers count on the drummer for not only the rhythms that animate their movement, but also for cues about when to perform certain context-dependent actions. Drumbeats provide energetic motivation for both kung fu and lion dance, but martial artists are inwardly focused during demonstrations in order to avoid following the drum, and dancers are much more outwardly attuned to the rhythms in order to entrain to them. Synchronization to the beat is doubly important when there is more than one lion. When there are two or more Hong Luck lions performing a routine together, they are in sync with each other through their entrainment to the percussion rhythms. They are also organized choreomusically by following cues from the drum so they start and end choreography at the same time.

In contrast, I observed several performances by lion dance troupes in Hong Kong where the lions were in time with the beat but out of sequence with one another. In these cases, one lion appeared to be the designated leader, initiating transitions between sections of choreography. It might have worked fine if it was a solo performance. With more than one lion, however, there was no way for the group to stay together. The drummer followed cues from the lead lion, and then the other lions tried to follow the drumming. The sonic transitions were abrupt as the drummer reacted to changes in choreography, which kept catching some of the other lion dancers off-guard and resulted in them being out of sync with the lead lion, the percussion, and one another. Luckily, what these performances lacked in entrainment they compensated for with flashy jumps and acrobatic tricks. Nonetheless, when I reported back to my teachers at Hong Luck about what I had seen, they criticized such unsynchronized performances as sloppy and undisciplined.

Their stance on entrainment and leadership in the lion dance pointed to a more martial understanding of choreomusical meanings.

Through martial sound, I interpret a synchronized relationship between drumming and lion dancing as embodying military order. Just as the soldiers of yore followed gong and drum signals from their generals, so do Hong Luck's martial lion dancers follow signals from drummers. Doing so allows the whole group to stay in time together, which is particularly important for multi-lion performances. That is not to say the drummer leads all the time; in some sections (like plucking-the-greens), the lion takes control of the choreomusical relationship. When my teachers disparaged lion-led performances as undisciplined, they revealed how they experience choreomusical relationships with, by means of, and through a martial body. Group entrainment in Hong Luck's lion dancing is desirable for the way it demonstrates embodied knowledge of, and skill in, a kung fu entrainment schema.

Inclusivity, Protention, and Leadership in Drumming

By 2014, I had begun to drum in public performances of both lion dance and kung fu. More skilled senior members were still the first choice to play the drum for important events, but I had proven my abilities sufficiently inside Hong Luck to be given more regular opportunities to play outside the club. Before getting into an interpretation of the experience of drumming martial sound, I will present an ethnographic vignette of what it was like playing the drum for the closing ceremony of the 2014 Chinatown Festival. Dundas Street West was closed to traffic for two full blocks east of Spadina Avenue, and throngs of people were strolling along, checking out the vendors, displays, food stalls, and entertainment. Over the Saturday and Sunday of that weekend, Hong Luck had put on multiple lion dance parades back and forth along the festival area, and we were finally making the last round.

It's nice doing a casual lion dance parade. The dancers are just mingling with the crowd, not performing rituals, and the choreography is all freestyle. The instruments are jamming on walking, side-to-side, and head-up beats, keeping the flow going. We have enough people to rotate all the positions, and so no one gets too tired. The weather is good, and everyone is feeling fine.

I'm playing the drum as we approach the main stage of the Chinatown Festival. Suddenly, a senior Hong Luck member starts to motion at us to wait. I shrug and continue drumming, but lower my volume, tempo, and variations down to a holding pattern while I wait to see what happens. Hearing the change in my beat, the lions stop moving forwards and hang out within earshot of the instruments.

The festival organizers get on stage and start making speeches in both Mandarin and Cantonese for the closing ceremony of the festival. I'm still not sure what we're doing here, so I split my attention among the speeches, the other instruments, and the lions. It's a bit tricky . . . when I play too quietly, the other instrumentalists can't follow my beat, but when I play too loudly, I can't hear the speeches. Meanwhile, the lions are loitering by the edge of the stage and mingling with passers-by. When the organizers thank Hong Luck, I momentarily increase my volume to cue three-bows, which the two lion dancers immediately respond to with the correct choreography. The MC then tells the crowd we will be regaled with a song, so I play a rhythmic cadence to halt the percussion. During the a cappella, someone comes over to tell us that we'll be doing a short lion dance on the stage after the singers are done.

I take a quick look to see who I'll be performing with. There are two current Hong Luck members under the lion heads and two older Hong Luck affiliates (kung fu masters in their own rights) playing gong and cymbals, all of whom are experienced performers. Nonetheless, we hadn't discussed a routine beforehand, so I make a mental note to use the clearest cues and most standard beats in order to make sure everyone can follow.

The two lions are ready by the side of the stage, and I start out strong with a head-up beat to signal them that it's time to begin. They quickly climb the short set of stairs and assume their positions at centre stage. Our crashing beats echo off the walls of the buildings lining the street and fill the air, but I'm a bit tired after an afternoon of parading . . . I'll have to be efficient if I'm going to make it through the performance at full volume. Thankfully, the gong and cymbal players are giving me plenty of sonic support.

I give three loud rim clicks to signal bows for the start of a freestyle routine, and then I go back to the head-up beat. The lion dancers shake their masks vigorously above their own heads until I give a powerful kung fu yell to mark a rhythmic cadence and cue three-rises. The gong player, cymbalist, and lion dancers are following well, and our energy is high. I play walking beats for a bit then reduce them to a quiet heartbeat as a transition to let everyone know we are moving on. When I see that the lions are waiting for my cue and hear the other instruments drop their volume in anticipation, I launch into a side-to-side beat. One lion is a bit slow to catch on, but both lions nail the crossover step at the end of it, which leads naturally back to walking. I switch to playing basic rhythms on "autopilot" as I scan the area to see if anyone has food for the lions. Once I've determined that there will be no eating, it's time to finish. Again, I yell to help cue three-rises, but this time I plan to add a sniff-the-tail rhythm to the end of it. When I see that both lion dancers are doing a knee-up three-rises that doesn't lead easily to sniff-the-trail, I abandon my plan and play a clean-the-beard rhythm instead. In the brief pause after the rhythmic cadence at the end of three-rises, I interject three rim clicks to let everyone know we aren't continuing with the routine, and then I play three-bows to end the performance.

A Hong Luck drummer's field of awareness encompasses more than that of the other performers. As the preceding description shows, I had to simultaneously be vigilant towards a number of contextual factors: the performance space, the audience/patrons, non-performing team members, the lion dancers, and the other instrumentalists. In the heat of performance, I felt my drumming being boosted by the gong and cymbals in order to completely fill the sonic space—even an outdoor one like Dundas Street West. Within the area defined by our martial sound, I was in control, but it still required a constant series of adjustments to keep everyone entrained to my beat. There is a delicate balance to playing fast and loud enough to both lead and encourage while also making continuous micro adjustments to timing that are reactive to the other performers and help everyone stay in the groove together.

In order to lead an inter-media lion dance performance, drummers must expand their focus to encompass a broader sense of the present moment. Dancers, cymbalists, and gong players, on the other hand, may tune into a narrower, more immediate instant as they follow the drummer. Music is one of Husserl's main examples in *Phenomenology of Internal Time Consciousness* (1964 [1928]), and his ideas help explain the experience of lion dance drumming. Husserl points out that our perception of "now" is not an instant where we experience only a single note at a time, but rather it is a now-moment, which can encompass a melody. Music can thus be fully experienced as music because of a broadened awareness of now's unfolding. I would add that the same thing happens with rhythm-based musicking. That is to say, one does not hear a string of single notes (individual instances of now) that must be actively reconstituted in memory; rather, one intuitively and immediately grasps them together as they unfold in time. To Husserl, music is immanent as a phenomenological object in the now-moment of time consciousness, which, I might add, is contingent upon the pre-reflexive cultural conditioning required to perceive a given span of humanly organized sound as music. In the expanded now-moment of musical experience, Husserl describes how retention keeps what has already passed connected to what is happening, while protention attaches what will happen next. This phenomenon is what allows both listeners and performers to perceive music as continuous, as opposed to a series of disjointed moments of sound.

Lion dance drummers use an expanded awareness of now to coordinate performances. A Hong Luck drummer, as the leader of the ensemble, controls the group's progression through a choreographed routine or determines an appropriate sequence for a freestyle performance. All members of the group have the same exposure to what has already happened, but the drummer's leading edge of protention is necessarily further into the future than the rest of the group. In the Chinatown Festival closing ceremony that I described, for example, I was the only person who actually knew what the next rhythm would be. While the other members of the group might have made educated guesses about what I would play, they still had to confirm and react when they heard it. As a lion dancer, there have been several times when I have forgotten parts of hastily choreographed routines and relied heavily on the drum to guide me. I have also occasionally been in performances where the drummer played something that was not part of the choreography, either by error or by choice, and I had no option but to follow along. Although drummers may have an idea of where they want to go with a freestyle routine, they must also be sensitive to unforeseen events that could change the direction of a performance, such as the agency of patrons or lion dancers, which adds an element of contingency to protention.

The onus is on the drummer to make or break a performance, and this can be especially challenging when there is a group of people performing lion dance who do not usually work together and/or have a wide range of different experience levels. Hong Luck members subscribe to the aesthetic that strong drumming can save a weak lion dance, but that poor drumming can ruin a good lion dance. Strong drumming does not mean just bashing away as loudly as possible or brazenly showing off one's skill, but rather playing in a way that makes the most of the ensemble members' differing abilities and pushes them to a level that they could not achieve without solid leadership. When I gained more experience behind the drum, I developed a greater appreciation for the value of Noah's straightforward style. It may not be as flashy as David's, but it is inclusive and easier for everybody to follow, and I try to emulate that in my own playing. That said, I prefer performing the lion dance with David as the drummer because his greater speed and power provide more energy. Even in set choreography, the rhythms are not over-determined and there is room for variation, so I value the way David mixes things up and presents challenges for me as a lion dancer. Additionally, his rhythmic virtuosity gives me more to work with in my movement. After David's drum lessons with Master Jim, he became more cognizant of the need to work within the abilities of the rest of his team. Nonetheless, he still likes to use his advanced technical ability to push the boundaries of performance, resulting in more exciting lion dances.

When a team of Hong Luck members work together regularly, especially when they are more skilled and/or experienced, the now-moment of performance can be more expansive. In such situations, the entrainment among drummer, gong player, cymbalists, head lion dancer(s), and tail lion dancer(s) is both tighter and more effortless. At that point, the dancers and supporting instruments are not just reacting to the drummer. Rather, their awareness expands to the point that rhythmic cues and cadences provide longer protention; they are thus better prepared for transitions, even when performing a freestyle routine. The result is an entrained togetherness manifested as seamless synchronization. It is in these situations that there is more room to actualize the extrinsic emotional content of a lion dance that Master Jim emphasized. When everyone is attuned to the structural foundation outlined by vocables, lion movement and drumming can more easily express emotion through intrinsic variations, embellishments, and spontaneity. For example, David enjoys being creative on the drum, but he can do his best drumming only when the rest of the group is in the groove and amplifying his energy.

Even when drummers focus their awareness on sound, movement is present in the drum rhythms. This indelible choreomusical connection is illustrated by Hong Luck members referring to the different types of beats in their repertoire according to the choreography they are associated with, a convention that I follow in my writing (e.g., bow, walking, head-up, three-rises).[1] The link between sound and movement is so strong that it persists in

---

[1] Many lion dance groups refer to rhythms and movements according to a star system that counts the number of notes and steps (Li 2017).

situations where the percussionists play without lion dancers. For instance, in the spring of 2014, David, Noah, and I were arranging Hong Luck's percussion repertoire for a recording that would be used in an award application. Notably, there would be no lion dancing in the recording because the award was music-centric. Our idea was to base the arrangement on the traditional lion dance routine but eliminate unnecessary repetition. My seniors told me they were having trouble conceiving of the sequence and flow of the beats without either dancing themselves or seeing someone dance it. We therefore proceeded to hash out the arrangement in terms of movement, working on the sequence of rhythm patterns through lion dance even though we only recorded the percussion part. Similarly, freestyle drumming, such as one might find before a parade or gig when the percussionists warm up the room, follows the general pattern of a lion dance including beginning and ending with three-bows. These examples show how Hong Luck members take a stance on drumming that is always-already in relationship to movement. The drum rhythms are the audile aspect of lion dancing even when there are no lions performing.

Some important aspects of drumming are internalized during training and are therefore not a focus during performance. A fundamental example is the absence of musical metre: there is no pattern of recurring strong and weak beats, and no regular length to the rhythmic cycles. Instead, kung fu and lion dance drumming styles use fairly even strength on pulses and their subdivisions, except for an emphasis on the last beat. When my cohort and I started learning to play the drum, we all unconsciously imposed a hierarchy of strong and weak beats characteristic of a 4/4 time signature. The percussion rhythms use duple subdivision, so our backgrounds in Western music likely conditioned us to feel them in what is called *common time*. Our misconception was particularly obvious in sections like the head-up or side-to-side that feature a string of eighth notes or quarter notes, respectively. It took some time and patience from my teachers to help me realize that the beats in these sections should be of equal strength, except for the emphasis on the last one. David suggested on several occasions that my drumming "sounds too much like reggae," by which he meant that I was emphasizing what would have been beats 2 and 4 in common time, as well as using slightly asymmetrical subdivisions that implied a swing feel. In class, David sought to correct my rhythmic deficiencies by coaching me to play continuous head-up beats "like a machine gun," as in fast but with motoric regularity. Similarly, Master Joe Kwong of the New Asia Kung Fu Society in Hong Kong taught

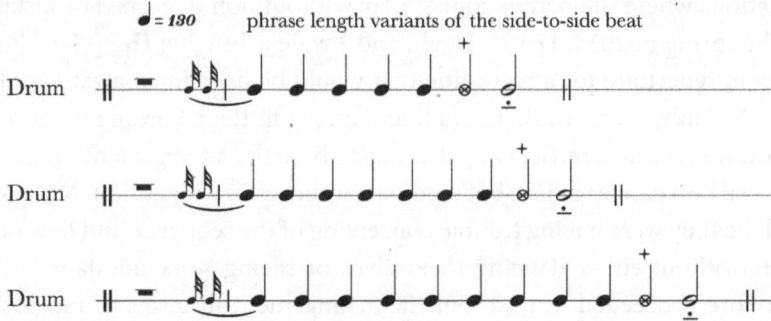

Figure 6.1 Side-to-side phrase length transcription
Credits: Colin P. McGuire

me to emphasize the last beat in a phrase rather than the first one, which he explained as being goal directed, driving towards the end of each phrase. At first, he had me over-exaggerate the final beat as an accent, but he later got me to ease off when I could emphasize the last beat in a more natural way.

Another characteristic of experiencing Hong Luck's martial sound is that the rhythmic structures are phrase based and the lengths of the phrases are variable. The traditional lion dance routine calls for variations of the side-to-side rhythm, for example, that could be seven, nine, or eleven beats long.[2] For drummers, phrase lengths are linked to the number of steps in a section of choreography, which forms the basis of their variability. The transcription in Figure 6.1 shows three different lengths of the side-to-side beat. All of them have a brief pickup and then a stream of quarter notes, which is the simplest version of this pattern. While drummers might vary the rhythms by using double-times, syncopations, and ornaments, the total length needs to remain the same in order to align with the choreography.

The variability of phrase lengths opens up interesting possibilities for improvisation when drumming is not directly linked to choreography. As previously mentioned, the walking beat is particularly amenable to variations and presents an opportunity for creating semi-improvised versions on the fly by combining, recombining, and/or altering patterns. A prime example of creative variation comes during lion dance parades when the default walking pattern can become tedious for all participants if the drummer keeps repeating

---

[2] Lion dancers' counting usually refers to the number of drum strokes but does not include rests or longer notes, i.e., a side-to-side beat with seven drum strokes covers eight beats' worth of time.

the same thing. The general structure of the walking drum pattern is loosely antiphonal; it is made up of cycles that alternate between a short root pattern as call and longer variations as answer. A basic pattern like the heartbeat (only two beats) would be played one or more times, and would then be answered by a pair of slightly longer variations (four beats each). The cycle begins anew with a return the short foundation rhythm. There is a wide variety of typical variations to choose from for the answer, which can further be elaborated by using rolls to fill in or replace beats, substituting drum strokes with mutes or rim clicks, and even spontaneously creating new rhythms that fit into the existing mould. The most extensive variations, however, happen when drummers manipulate phrase length to extend the answer rhythms, creating opportunities for surprising recombinations.

When I am drumming, I experience extension of a phrase as keeping the beat "up," whereas a "down" beat would feel like the emphasis that marks the end of a phrase. The feeling of being up is one that maintains rhythmic energy to give the impression of continuous forward movement. By withholding the emphasis that marks the final beat, I open the door to being able to link rhythms together, repeat patterns, and even draw in partial references to non-walking beats. A more advanced drummer like David seems to be able to extend his variations almost indefinitely, which he fills in with more elaborate rolls, mutes, and rim clicks. Extending phrases during free variation is tricky, however, because there is room for accents, syncopations, and pauses that function as participatory discrepancies to create a feel or groove (Keil 1987), without necessarily having the structural significance of a final beat. Furthermore, the emphasis that signals finality is not about playing significantly louder or harder as an accent, but rather delivering a weighted beat that brings the phrase down to a close.

In reflecting on the experience of phrase extension, it became evident that sound was less important than silence in marking the end of a pattern, but that there was also a physical component. In the brief pause after a final beat, there is a momentary release of sonic tension. Nonetheless, not all rests have the same effect because a mute in the middle of a phrase does not indicate finality. Varying phrase length in lion dance drumming relies on the ability not only to maintain the energy of a passage (to keep it "up"), but also to finalize the phrase with an emphatic pause after the downbeat (to let it "down"). The trick with emphasizing the last beat is that the silence following it is active. David has tried to explain to me the energy of the pause after a final beat as non-stopping, leaving a space that is active by its inactivity. His explanations came across as a bit philosophical or poetic until I experienced how it works in performance with other people. As experienced, one punctuates rhythm patterns with an emphasis on the last beat but turns them into phrases by playing silence after the final sound. Active inactivity means stopping phys-ical motion while maintaining dynamic physical tension, pausing in a way that entrains the gong and cymbal players to the phrase's end. In that mo-ment, silence and stillness combine as drummers momentarily sink deeper into the horse stance, bringing the beat down through a stance of finality.

Conclusion

The current chapter has provided thick, phenomenological descriptions of Hong Luck's practices as cases studies to demonstrate the embodied understandings I outlined in the previous chapter. In order to fold these two chapters together, here is a brief recap of a few key points from Chapter 5. I discussed my teacher Noah's belief that the most appreciative audiences for Hong Luck's martial sound are kung fu and/or lion dance practitioners, as well as people with a lifetime of experience with these practices. I then considered how embodiment could provide a framework for understanding the meaning of this type of percussion musicking. In writing about African music, John Chernoff has suggested that "[m]ovement is the key to 'hearing' the music" (1979: 22), and I argue that this is also the case with Hong Luck's percussion. My discussion of embodied hearing proceeded along two intertwined lines of inquiry: uncovering practitioners' experience through the body in order to give non-practitioners a ground for understanding, and the various ways an entrainment schema provides the basis of metaphorical meanings.

Hong Luck's martial sound emanates from a body of ideas related to mil-itary drill, the rhythm of combat, and battlefield signals, and it expresses choreomusical meanings through the relationships of sound and movement. While gong and drum percussion ensembles are found in Chinese ritual, op-eratic, and festive traditions more broadly (Jones 1995), the diasporic context in Canada has diluted these broader associations while strengthening kung fu connections. Additionally, martial arts seek to engrain combative rhythms into the bodies of practitioners. By hearing fighting skills musically, I flipped the post-structuralist tendency to read meaningful action as text and/or dis-course. Not to overemphasize the martial, I also engaged with Master Jim's fourfold approach to understanding lion dance. His choreomusical view gathered sound, movement, structure, and emotion to present meaning in action.

In this chapter, I delved more deeply into the experience of performing kung fu, lion dance, and drumming. Longer, first-person, ethnographic vignettes aimed to reveal the scope of a performer's awareness and the entrainment relationships between sound and movement. More specifically, I showed how martial arts demos require a narrow focus that allows performers to hear the percussion—but not heed it—in order to maintain an asynchronous relationship to the beats. This choreomusical relationship evokes the rhythm of combat while drawing on sonic motivation from the percussion. I explained how lion dancers have a medium focus because the mask limits their vision, forcing them to entrain their movements to the drummer's beat. They rely on drum signals to orient them like troops on a battlefield, which helps compensate for their visual deficiency. Through martial sound, lion dancers know when to enact choreography and how to stay in sync with one another. The final vignette showed how drummers maintain a multi-sensory awareness of both the performance context and fellow performers in order to orchestrate the proceedings but remain responsive to unforeseen changes. I closed my interpretation with considerations of where performers fit into the now-moment of musical time, showing how flexible phrasing in Hong Luck's drumming allows drummers to manipulate structure during performance.

In this chapter I have relied extensively on my own perspective as a practitioner of Hong Luck's kung fu, lion dance, and percussion in order to present and interpret how these arts are given in experience. In Chinese culture, it is considered rude to boast, and even accepting compliments can be seen as impolite, so I would like to make it clear that my performance ethnography in no way implies a claim of mastery. Nonetheless, I am on solid ground in claiming my experiences to be legitimate because Hong Luck has recognized my embodied knowledge. I was honoured to be nominated and approved by the board of the Hong Luck Association as an official lion dance team leader, including having my Chinese name [*Mahkgwāi Gōlìhn*, 麥桂歌連][3] published alongside the list of other Hong Luck officials in a local Chinese

---

[3] My Chinese name is a transliteration of my English one. The second character of my surname has at times been transcribed differently as either "cassia, laurel, or cinnamon" [*gwai*, 桂] or "sundial or ceremonial jade tablet" [*gwāi*, 圭], both of which are homophonous except for their tone. The former is probably more appropriate because it is also a Chinese surname.

newspaper. I was also honoured when Master Jim asked me to assist him in teaching the advanced kung fu class, and Noah let me teach lion dance class without supervision. I write the above to show that my kung fu, lion dance, and drumming abilities have been approved by both seniors and elders at the club. The unfathomable interiority of being-in-the-world means that I cannot claim my experiences to be equivalent to those of my consultants. Nonetheless, they have confirmed that I am experiencing their practices with, by means of, and through the same things that they are.

This chapter has provided an interpretation of the embodied meanings of Hong Luck's martial sound as both combative rhythms and percussion musicking. The interdisciplinary nature of kung fu as a blurred genre means that movement is always present in martial sound—even when the instrumentalists play on their own (i.e., without accompanying other performers). Practitioners experience martial sound through choreomusical relationships engrained by training in martial arts and lion dance. Their perception of the drumming is both functional and visceral; the drum rhythms frame, structure, and organize performance while also energizing the performers. Informed audiences are more likely to have an ideomotor (mental) experience of Hong Luck's martial sound, rather than practitioners' sensorimotor (embodied) one (Reybrouck 2001), but both perceive the relationship of sound to movement, and can thus hear the movement in the sound. Following Mark Johnson's (1987, 1997) ideas about meaning and embodied metaphor, I have proposed a previously unnamed image schema for discussing Hong Luck's martial sound. More specifically, I contend that an entrainment schema undergirds meaning in performances of kung fu and lion dance: the struggle of martial artists to remain asynchronous from the beats is characteristic of the rhythm of combat; lion dancers' reliance on drum cues brings a military quality to their ritual; and drummers' multifaceted role in performance positions them as generals who motivate, give signals, and impose the club's sonic will on the performance space. In the next, and final, chapter, I summarize my findings and provide an integrated view of the multivalent meanings of Hong Luck's blurred genre. I also consider the club's future, including the challenges it faces going into its sixth decade.

7

Bringing the Past into the Future

Introduction

At the start of this book, I stated that my objective was to investigate how movement and sound work together in kung fu in order to reveal their role in empowering a resilient, diasporic, community identity. I then proposed the concept of *martial sound* for hearing all aspects of human combative behaviour. My objective, and the theory I developed for it, was purposefully broad, because my aim has been to contribute to broader discussions about community, diaspora, and embodiment in relation to sonic being-in-the-world. Nonetheless, it was potentially misleading to imply that there could be an all-encompassing relationship between movement and sound, that kung fu as a blurred genre could be reduced to a single purpose, or that a diasporic Chinese martial arts group is part of a single, clearly defined community. On the contrary, my research shows that the very potency of martial sound is found in the multiplicity of its expressions and diverse meanings. Throughout this book, my ethnography has focused on describing, explaining, analysing, and interpreting the practices of the Hong Luck Kung Fu Club in all their diversity. In this conclusion, I do not attempt to collapse my findings into uniformity. Instead, I revisit the pieces as part of a holistic mosaic whose dynamic synergy can be better appreciated as a multi-vocal, multifaceted, multivalent whole.

The luxury of time is probably the best thing about doing fieldwork close to home (Stock and Chou 2008 [1997]). In my case, it allowed me to learn Hong Luck's drumming according to the painstaking traditional transmission process. After six years of fieldwork, my doctoral research and dissertation for this project was complete, but I trained at the club for another two years. I then left Toronto, but I continued revising, augmenting, and expanding the research for this book, which took another couple of years. In many ways, however, my work with Hong Luck's practices has only just begun. In the course of my training I became a member of Hong Luck's overlapping communities in a much more permanent way than I could have imagined.

Martial Sound. Colin P. McGuire, Oxford University Press. © Oxford University Press 2024.
DOI: 10.1093/oso/9780197775936.003.0007

The fieldwork may technically be done, but I cannot simply leave the "field." The long-term, intensive nature of the process has made the field a state of being rather than simply a place. I am not alone in this embedded-ness. Most of the club's senior members have expressed feelings of camaraderie and obligation that have kept them coming back to Hong Luck. Moreover, the practices of kung fu, lion dance, and percussion embed people in martial, ritual, artistic, and musical communities of practice through doing that leads to becoming. Hong Luck members remain part of the club—even if they are no longer regular participants on the training floor—through embodied and sonic legacies that live on at the club.

My fieldwork was done at a transitional time in Hong Luck's history, when the future of the club had come into question for several reasons. Foremost among these was the passing of co-founding Masters Paul Chan in 2012 and Jim Chan in 2016, but changing social interest in—and valuation of—traditional martial arts has also loomed large. The time is therefore ripe to disseminate more information about the importance of old-school Southern Chinese martial arts, for not only practitioners but also their local and trans-national communities. In particular, I want to emphasize how kung fu, as a holistic blurred genre, offers flexible pathways of becoming within the stream of tradition. In this conclusion, I review the findings of my research at the intersection of sound, movement, and meaning. First, I summarize how martial sound fits into kung fu as a blurred genre in the realms of community and empowerment. Next, I discuss the legacy of the club's founders and the future of Hong Luck's traditions. Finally, I consider the implications of sound and music in the study of martial arts more generally.

Empowering the Community: Sound, Movement, and Meaning

Rhythm is at the heart of the Hong Luck Kung Fu Club, from the long cycle of annual events to the weekly schedule of training (Blue 2014), and from the choreomusical patterns of lion dance rituals to the arrangements of martial sound in kung fu class. Drumming is the club's heartbeat. As audile lifeblood, Hong Luck's percussive martial sound circulates, sustains, and enlivens. By augmenting the typical benefits of martial arts training (e.g., fitness, discipline, self-defence), drumming helps diverse communities adhere and makes various forms of resistance audible.

Hong Luck's communities spread out in overlapping, concentric circles. The inner circle is the community of practice developed through training in kung fu as a blurred genre. The beginner class initiates muscular bonding, which is deepened by the teamwork of the lion dance troupe, through the agonic fellowship of sparring partners, and with the pseudo-kinship network that structures the club's social hierarchy. Long-term participation establishes bonds of friendship, too, particularly when members sometimes spend more time with one another at the club than they do outside with friends or families. For the lion dance team especially, camaraderie is built not only while training and performing, but also at the customary post-gig dinners. The next circle is the local Chinatown community. As I described in Chapter 3, performing lion dance, percussion, and kung fu allows Hong Luck members to fulfil social roles in Chinatown, regardless of whether they live there, have Chinese heritage, or speak Chinese. As a ritual, lion dance auspicates new beginnings and calendric events by driving away negative energy to make room for good things like luck, happiness, and prosperity. It is also a performance of Chinese identity at events and festivals. Through twice-yearly parades, lion dancing is an active patrol by which Hong Luck claims the Spadina/Dundas area as Chinatown's space. Martial sound fuels both ritual efficacy and performative entertainment, extending the lion(s)'s sphere of influence to the farthest reaches of hearing, and announcing Hong Luck's presence as an integral part of the community.

The biggest circle of Hong Luck's communities is the "martial forest" [*móuh làhm*, 武林], as kung fu subculture is known. Once secretive and confined to the margins of society in China, kung fu has gradually become a transnational community of practitioners—and audiences. Whereas Chinese martial arts have long appeared in street performances, opera, storytelling, and serialized novels in China, modern technology and transnational flows have greatly expanded opportunities for audience engagement. Kung fu is now practised and appreciated in all corners of the world. The opening up of Chinese martial subculture has extended the community by allowing people from all walks of life to practise traditional martial arts and lion dance, as well as to enjoy kung fu cultural products such as movies, videos, television, opera, literature, competitions, blogs, and gaming. Notwithstanding rivalries between different styles, schools, or practitioners of kung fu (and their fans), being a part of the twenty-first-century Chinese martial arts community means having the subcultural and/or embodied knowledge to participate in a somewhat esoteric, formerly marginal, but now transnational, subculture.

In the City of Toronto, where the official civic motto since 1997 has been "Diversity: Our Strength," Hong Luck's Chinese-ness is an interesting case study of how inclusion can work in a multicultural community. Not that "Chinese" itself is a stable, straightforward, or uncontested category; there are distinctions to be made between nationalist, linguistic, ethnic, and regional variations of what the term means. For example, Hong Luck's founders were from Guangdong Province, as were a majority of Chinese Canadians up until the late twentieth century, but Chinatown now has people from other parts of Greater China and the diaspora, speaking a variety of Sinitic languages and living divergent versions of Chinese culture. Nonetheless, Hong Luck is distinctly Chinese in a way that includes, rather than excludes, which I can illustrate with a further example. During Chinese New Year 2014, the Consul General of China visited Hong Luck Upstairs to pay his respects, and I was invited to attend along with a group of senior members. He commended the elders for their sustained impact on promoting Chinese culture in diaspora, commenting that it is important for Chinese Canadians to continue loving China while also embracing Canada. Since its early days, the club has had an inclusive stance—admitting people of all backgrounds— and the Consul General also approvingly acknowledged that kung fu is a good way of introducing non-Chinese Canadians to Chinese culture. Much to the Consul General's satisfaction, Hong Luck's president remarked that the club has non-Chinese members like me (among others) who have even been inspired to learn some Chinese. As I discussed in Chapter 4, Master Paul explicitly demanded the embodiment of Chinese-ness in the club's martial arts. The club's founders, Hong Luck's president, and the Consul General all welcomed and encouraged kung fu practitioners of any cultural, ethnic, or national background, which points to their stance on inclusivity in the diasporic Chinese community through embodied being.

Claiming the idea of cultural China (i.e., the Sino-sphere of Chinese peoples, not just the PRC) as an inclusive, transnational community is a strategy of what political scientist Joseph Nye calls *soft power* (1990). Notably, the opportunity to embody Chinese-ness beyond the geo-political boundaries of the PRC, including for people of other citizenships, nationalities, and ethnicities, is more than a short-term or limited tactic. As compared to the temporary nature of what postcolonial theorist Gayatri Spivak's terms *strategic essentialism* (1988), where subaltern groups gloss over the differences of their constituents to represent a basic shared identity when mobilizing for specific political ends, Chinese-ness is a more durable construct. Kung fu

as soft power contributes to building global goodwill through attraction, interest, and appeal, rather than the coercive resources of military force and economic pressure that make up hard power. That is to say, soft power renders
other cultures and nations positively disposed towards cultural China, thus
providing cultural capital to Chinese people and facilitating their endeavours
in many aspects of life. The Chinese-ness of kung fu still relies on a strategy
of cultural essence, so I propose that it extends strategic essentialism into the
more stable realm of soft power, as well as helping to create a sort of transnational imagined community (Anderson 2006 [1983]; McGuire 2018) that
is not limited to citizens of the PRC. Whether in the emergent habitus of
practitioners or the media dreams of audiences, Chinese martial arts are an
engaging point of entry and return to cultural China. Notably, martial sound
helps give voice to people who would embody Chinese-ness, but do not
speak Chinese. The ability to play kung fu percussion instruments and/or
generate sound through martial arts allows those who do not speak Chinese
to express themselves sonically in a Chinese way.

As much as kung fu contributes to empowered community building and
wields soft power, it is still a martial art capable of literally resisting violence.
Hong Luck members consider hand combat skills to be fundamental to all
of their performance practices. In performance, lion dancers and martial
artists show their strength, dexterity, and skill with heroic displays of pre-
paredness for self-defence. The gong and drum ensemble that accompanies
performances amplifies the impact of martial motion and is also itself a pres-
entation of warriors' expertise. For outsiders, such demonstrations might
be an opaque cultural expression, although certainly an interesting and
colourful one. For insiders, kung fu's blurred genre is a stance on the heroic "martial virtue" [*móuh dāk*, 武德] of the Shaolin Temple and anti-Qing
revolutionaries. Trained fighters in Toronto's Chinatown community have,
through their public presence, bolstered the morale of Chinese people who
have been subject to institutional and social racism. Sometimes empowering
performances are not enough, however, and many Hong Luck members
have stories about having had to use their fighting skills in racially motivated
confrontations. Street fighting to defend oneself, community, property,
and honour is less common than it used to be, but it remains a necessity in
Toronto to this day. When soft power fails, kung fu's hard power abides.

More recently, lion dance has become an arena for a different kind of
empowerment. Due to the traditional exclusion of women from all but
supporting roles, lion dancing's purported masculinity has contributed to

unequal constructions of gender, ability, and power. Now that women have begun to lion dance at Hong Luck, they are taking an embodied stance on a new type of power that shows their strength and challenges patriarchal claims to exclusive civil and martial authority. Eventually, females will become drummers at Hong Luck, which will sound empowerment in thunderous ways.

Finally, Hong Luck's adherence to tradition represents a stance on resisting the vagaries of a rapidly changing world. Tradition is never truly static, and traditional Chinese martial arts avoid breaking with the past by maintaining continuity of change and preserving intangible cultural heritage. In an interesting twist, a new generation of female lion dancers are taking up the torch of Hong Luck's lion dance with traditional martial vigour, maintaining the core of the ritual efficacy even while transgressing previous gender limitations.

Lineage and Legacy Following the Death of Masters

In November 2013, filmmaker Diana Dai shot a segment at Hong Luck for her documentary on Toronto's Chinatown.[1] When she interviewed Master Jim Chan, who was the head instructor at the time, she asked him about his hopes for the club's future. He replied, "I hope they will teach what I taught them" [*ngóh hēimòhng kéuihdeih wúi gaau ngóh gaau-jó kéuihdeih ge jeh*, 我希望佢地會教我教咗佢地嘅嘢]. She pressed him to elaborate, but Master Jim simply reiterated, "if they teach what I taught them, that's enough" [*yuhgwó kéuihdeih gaau ngóh gaau-jó kéuihdeih ge jeh, jauh dāk la*, 如果佢地教我教咗佢地嘅嘢就得啦]. Hong Luck's co-founder was succinctly referring to the club's entire half-century legacy of kung fu, lion dance, and martial sound, including the repertoire of several styles of kung fu, which will be no mean feat to preserve and transmit to the next generation.

The liminal moment of generational turnover upon the death of a master is a rich—albeit sad—time for (re)examining how the past, present, and future of a community of practice are imagined. When a tradition-bearer reaches an advanced age, the issue of his/her legacy is thrust into the forefront of consciousness for the next generation. It is thus an opportune time for an ethnographer to observe how people grapple directly with matters that are often unconscious in day-to-day practice. My ethnography of the Hong Luck

---

[1] *Crossing Chinatown* http://www.dianadai.com/9.html.

Kung Fu Club revealed telling group discourses about tradition and change when long-time head instructor Master Paul passed. After Master Jim took over the mantle of head instructor, but just prior to his passing, my personal relationship with him as his disciple made me privy to his concerns about the fragility of body-experience and the ways that an embodied legacy is preserved through lineage transmission. The loss felt at the passing of these octogenarian head instructors was exacerbated by the diasporic situation. The masters represented a living cultural connection with a historical China that now only exists in memory and imagination. Furthermore, the intangible nature of oral, aural, and embodied lineage highlighted the contingency of transmission. Authentically re-inventing a tradition may be more significant to embodied legacies than faithful copying, paradoxically using change as a tool for conservation.

I contend that legacies of cultural expression essentially form a guided re-invention of a master's embodied experience. To understand them in this way adds a layer of nuance to discourses of tradition preservation. While "legacy" and "tradition" are sometimes used interchangeably, they are by no means exact equivalents. Differentiating these two concepts will help me explain the legacies of Hong Luck's two co-founding masters. More broadly, I hope to shed light on how the deeply personal aspects of body-experience lineage do not simply represent the past; they also enliven the present and endow the future. First, I differentiate between tradition and legacy, next I summarize the situation at Hong Luck, then I discuss Master Jim's legacy, and I finish with a case study on tensions surrounding reproduction versus creativity in martial sound.

Tradition, Legacy, and Lineage

Before continuing, I need to clarify some terminology, starting with my use of the words *legacy* and *tradition* in this section. Both refer to things that are handed down, but they are not wholly synonymous. *Tradition* implies customs, practices, and/or beliefs that are longstanding in nature and have been passed on through generations. In theory, Hobsbawm and Ranger (1983) have thoroughly problematized the invented nature of many allegedly "ancient" traditions, but in practice the word still suggests conservation of old ways. Of course, cultural expressions rarely stay the same as they are passed along, so continuity of change is more likely than exact replication. Tradition also has a collective quality because it is sustained by groups of people over time. As James Kippen has observed of *ustāds* and their disciples in the tablā tradition of North India, "[t]he maintenance of tradition as a shared body of skills and knowledge therefore requires . . . active links in the chain of musical transmission: at least three generations are held to be necessary for the chain to have structural integrity" (Kippen 2008 [1997]: 127).

Legacy, on the other hand, typically refers to something passed down from a specific predecessor. Such predecessors are known entities, rather than the types of anonymous, collective, or semi-mythical origins of many traditions. The historicity of legacy contrasts with the implied timelessness of tradition. Legacy also has legal and technical connotations. In law, a legacy is a bequest of property or money after someone dies. In technology, legacy is an adjective describing hardware or software that continues to be used even though it is no longer supported by its creators. In the realm of cultural expression, legacy bears the traces of legal and technological meanings, connoting a predecessor's inheritance that is valuable despite not being current.

Hong Luck members recognize Master Paul's legacy as the club itself, but Master Jim's contribution is less tangible—though no less important. The two co-founders are like yin and yang. Master Paul was equal parts statesman and warrior, leveraging his diverse social, economic, cultural, and political connections to build Hong Luck, while undergirding the club's practice with his fighting ability. In contrast, Master Jim was much more internally focused. He used to tell me that he looked after the technical side of kung fu, whereas Master Paul was the public face, the leader, and the fighter. Master Jim focused primarily on enhancing Hong Luck's martial excellence through attention to detail on the training floor and its expression in performance, and he was relatively less concerned with politics or social standing. To be sure, their roles as kung fu instructors overlapped, but their legacies are divergent.

Looking Back, Looking Forward: Tradition in Toronto, Then and Now

Over the course of this book, I have mentioned a number of factors that have put Hong Luck's legacy on shifting ground. I revisit these here in a consideration of the club's future. As compared to the situation of racial exclusion when the club was founded, Chinese Canadians are now more accepted in

Canada's multicultural mosaic. Moreover, China has risen to global prominence as a superpower. The combination of these first two factors means that there is less need for self-defence, and tong associations are no longer essential to survival of Chinese Canadians. When it comes to the physical culture of martial arts, the tides have also shifted. After Bruce Lee ushered in the kung fu craze of the 1970s (Bowman 2013), Hong Luck's training hall was filled past capacity with eager students looking for Chinese martial arts. That era was also a golden age for traditional lion dancing, thanks to a deep network of community support and limited competition from other kung fu clubs. While martial arts have continued to accrue public interest on an international scale, it is now MMA that rules the spotlight, thanks in large part to the media-savvy efforts of the Ultimate Fighting Championship (UFC). Similarly, the acrobatics of competition-style lion dance and the flashiness of modern wushu performance have eclipsed the traditional kung fu styles of groups like Hong Luck. These various factors have converged, and now the club struggles to get enough income from tuition, gigs, and donations to keep the doors open.

The fiftieth anniversary in 2011 and Master Paul Chan's death in 2012 were milestones that prompted discussions among Hong Luck's membership about the club's status and its future. These two events attracted many senior members who were no longer regularly active at the club, but who enriched the conversations with their experiences from decades gone by. During the year of the fiftieth anniversary, people were generally respectful and complimentary, as was befitting such a celebration. Despite all due respect for Hong Luck's half-century of preserving and promoting Chinese kung fu in Canada, several returning senior members hinted at disappointment that the club was not what they remembered it to be. While nostalgia certainly played a role in their qualitative evaluations, there has been a quantifiable decrease in students and lion dance gigs.

Notably, Hong Luck alumni with successful clubs of their own have departed in various ways from the inherited traditions of their teachers.[2] These departures include focusing exclusively on kickboxing, changing Hong Luck's forms to make them more crowd-pleasing, mixing kung fu with personal fitness training, and embracing competition-style lion dancing. In

---

[2] Martial arts schools in the Greater Toronto Area operated by Hong Luck alumni include: Northern Leg Southern Fist, JV Martial Arts Studio, Bamboo Kung Fu, Sammy Cheng Toronto Lion Dance Association, Twin Dragon Kung Fu and Kickboxing Club, and Body by Dex.

the wake of Master Paul's death, leaders from several of these offshoot clubs tried to suggest changes to Hong Luck that would "improve" the curriculum, which the remaining elders and the active seniors soundly rejected.

When co-founding Master Jim Chan came out of retirement in 2012 to take up the vacant position of head instructor, he reinforced Hong Luck's mandate as a bastion of tradition. On his watch, there was even a reactionary shift towards an older, village-style of Choi Lee Fut, rather than the mainstream variety that Master Paul had been promoting near the end of his life. Unfortunately, Master Jim's return to active duty was not enough to fully revitalize the club. In November 2013, a senior member who had been at the club for over thirty years characterized the situation to me with a lion metaphor: "We don't roar anymore. It's just a whisper . . . just a meow."

Master Jim's passing in the fall of 2016 was the end of an era and the beginning of a long liminal moment for Hong Luck. The club's remaining elders and the senior instructors nominated Master Paul's son-in-law to become the next head instructor; this provided some continuity, as he was a disciple of both the founders. The position is mostly honorary, however, and my consultants tell me that the new "head instructor" is barely involved in the club's day-to-day affairs. Furthermore, Hong Luck Upstairs gradually reduced and eliminated its tong activities, which used to be an important source of both income and administrative oversight. Hong Luck is currently being stewarded by a committee of senior members. With a younger generation in charge of the club, the question of continuity versus change looms large.

When I caught up with several of the key instructors and administrators in October 2018, they explained how the club is still grappling with how to reconcile past, present, and future. They told me they have been trying to maintain Hong Luck's traditions, but that an ad hoc approach to the status quo is leading to gradual decay. They expressed concerns about how best to preserve the legacy of Master Paul's vision for Hong Luck: as a node in a transnational community of kung fu practice; as a centre for traditional Chinese culture in diaspora; and as a hub in the local Chinatown connecting tong associations, businesses, Chinese Canadians, and non-Chinese Canadians. The problem is how to honour that legacy through traditional blurred genre kung fu while continuing to be relevant in a rapidly changing world. Now that the Hong Luck Upstairs tong has ceased operations, the second floor of the building is being rented out for extra income, which has provided a financial cushion and support for continuing to teach traditional kung fu without bowing to market pressures. Nonetheless, changes are being tested to make the curriculum more appealing to potential students, such as allowing them to fast-track into the lion dance or sparring classes.

Master Jim's Legacy and the Reinvention of Tradition

I trained intensely with Master Jim in his final years, when he was urgently trying to secure the continuity of his own distinct lineage, which was less well represented at Hong Luck because of Master Paul's long prominence as head instructor. Two weeks before Master Jim passed away, he told me that I was his best student. He did not mean I was the most talented or the best practitioner, because he recognized the martial and musical abilities of other students as being better than mine. For example, he referred to David as a kung fu "genius" [*tīnchòih*, 天才]. What Master Jim meant was that I had learned from him with the most keenness and fidelity, which I attribute to my methodological approach of using apprenticeship as ethnography. A key example has to do with the Taishan walking beats that Master Jim taught David, and that I learned as an observer of the lessons. David already had a well-developed personal style, and he told me he was not particularly en-thusiastic about Master Jim's traditional beats. David dutifully learned the Taishan walking rhythms, but he treated them more as an exercise than as repertoire. I, on the other hand, have taken an ethnomusicologist's glee in this rare drumming style, and so I have endeavoured to play it in public when-ever possible. I was also delighted when Master Jim reinvented the Dragon Boxing form that I described in Chapter 6, which he did using my body as a canvas. He conceded that he could not remember the exact sequence of moves, and thus needed to fill in some gaps, but he also told me that the form he gave me still had the unique character that tradition required. The last time I saw him, Master Jim proudly said my kung fu (in the broad sense) had become the same as his master, and that his work was thus done. I now find myself implicated in the chain of transmission, because my master made me promise I would teach what he taught me.

Master Jim was acutely aware of the need to pass on his personal embodied knowledge, not just the formal aspects of kung fu movement and sound. In contradistinction to the widely shared tradition of Southern Chinese kung fu in general, and Choi Lee Fut in particular, I am referring to our master's way of being-in-the-world through kung fu. It is here that legacy separates from tradition in that Master Jim was more concerned with how we did kung fu than he was with dogmatic reproduction of choreography, technique, or rhythm. He told me that his Choi Lee Fut was inflected by his study of Northern Sect [*Bāk Paai*, 北派] kung fu, which he explained was more acrobatic, exaggerated, and theatrical than Southern styles. Through this influence, Master Jim developed a highly refined method of performing violence. Senior students noted that our teacher had changed some of the sequences in choreographed forms over time, but that he always insisted on particular ways of doing kung fu, to which I will return. While some changes to choreography may have been due to failing memory (which Master Jim freely admitted), in other cases it was more that the choreography was fungible and less important than the embodied knowledge being expressed. At the conclusion of one form, for example, students in my class were doing at least three different movement sequences for the final combination, and Master Jim said it was all fine as long as it had the right embodied character. Moreover, our teacher gave extensive coaching on the performative qualities of Master Paul's forms, showing that his legacy was equally applicable to a parallel tradition of martial arts.

To explain what Hong Luck's head instructor was focused on teaching, I draw on the concept of *body-experience lineage*, as developed by sociologist and physical education scholar David Brown (2014). Brown argues that a master's bodily capital continues to live in the bodies of his/her students, and so corporeal knowledge is at risk of being lost if it is not transmitted. Traditional practices like martial arts, dance, and music may be documented and preserved through various forms of recording and notation, but body-experience exceeds the audio-visual. When it is handed down to the next generation, it creates a somatic lineage such that part of the master lives on in the disciple. Intersubjective processes of teaching, learning, and training allow a master to transmit their sense of feel and their practical logic through shared kinaesthesia.

At Hong Luck, I experienced the transmission of body-experience as Master Jim coached me in a process of (re)discovery. Noted mathematician Hans Freudenthal calls this style of teaching and learning *guided reinvention* (1991). The idea is that, rather than prescribing reified models or focusing on rote learning, teachers guide their students through experiential processes of rediscovering the material for themselves. Freudenthal writes, "the learner should reinvent mathematising rather than mathematics" (1991: 49), and Master Jim asked us to reinvent kung fu-ing rather than kung fu. Master Jim attempted to guide us students towards a personal rediscovery of the experiences that had shaped his body-knowledge as a martial artist. In addition to the timing and rhythms that I have discussed elsewhere, he was particularly concerned with force and intentionality. Master Jim often repeated phrases (in both English and Cantonese) such as "hand and horse (stance) together" [*sáu tùhng máh yāt chàih*, 手同馬一齊], "good kung fu needs eyes" [*hóu gūngfū yiu ngáahn*, 好功夫要眼], and "you must use your mind" [*néih yiu séung*, 你要想]. He was not simply repeating these things for lack of something "more" to teach or from the mental frailty of old age, as some of my classmates told me in private that they feared. On the contrary, Master Jim confided in me that he kept saying these maxims because students still needed to work on them. He was pointing to the keys that would unlock rediscovery of his body-experience, but it was up to students to open the door. Our teacher wanted to see real fighting power in choreographed forms coming from full bodily coordination; he wanted to feel bloodlust in our eyes showing full commitment to martial self-expression; and he wanted us to use our minds to manifest an invisible opponent, making our demonstrations more than just Shaolin shadowboxing.

Finally, Master Jim wanted to hear us express martial sound over top of the extreme loudness of the percussion ensemble during demonstrations. He repeatedly admonished students that the yells used to punctuate the ends of striking combinations were never loud enough, fearsome enough, or lusty enough. The term he used was *giu sēng* [叫聲], implying the type of yell an animal would make; he wanted us to roar like lions. Some students may not have had the physical capacity to project their voices that loudly, but many of the junior students also appeared to be too timid to bellow at the top of their lungs. Like the *kiai* [気合] of Japanese martial arts, a powerful yell in kung fu can be used as martial sound to startle or intimidate an opponent and to bolster one's own confidence, all while tightening the muscles of the abdomen to withstand a counterattack. In some styles of Choi Lee Fut, such as mainstream Hung Sing as promoted by Master Paul, there are specific vocable sounds attached to certain types of techniques. There are three main vocables shouted when executing the following moves: kicks are *dīk* [嘀], tiger claws are *wāa* [嘩], and ginger fist (a.k.a. panther paw) punches are *yīk* [嘀]. In Master Jim's village-style Choi Lee Fut, however, there are no required words or syllables. Instead, the goal is a primal scream. When he came out of retirement to assume the mantle of Hong Luck's head instructorship, Master Jim no longer had the strength to shout loudly, but he still demonstrated the

roar with a bloodcurdling sonic quality. In the summer of 2016, I was starting
to get the right timbre; one needs to engage both primary and false vocal
chords, as is done in some types of throat singing and in heavy-metal vocals.
Confirmation came as I was practising a kung fu form and gave a particularly
lion-like roar. Master Jim commented to one of the other elders within earshot of the class, "his vocal tone is good" [*kéuih háuhei hóu hóu*, 佢口氣好
好], and, appropriately, the term *háuhei* [口氣] literally means *mouth energy*,
although David teased me that the slang meaning is *bad breath*.

I contend that experiencing reinvention is integral to preserving a master's
intangible legacy, and that lineage transmission is about more than just
technique. While intangible, Master Jim's legacy is powerful because of his
particular way of coordinating mind and body to manifest fighting spirit
in performance. All fighting arts involve the coordination of mental and
physical faculties to generate power; but the subtleties of gesture, timing,
and intention combine to create a martial way of being-in-the-world that is
as unique as a fingerprint. Just doing the movements correctly is thus not
enough, and only lineage holders can confirm that a student has embodied
the experience. Transmission is intersubjectively confirmed when a master
can see themselves in the student. To reach that point, much bodily information is transmitted through touch, as when a master nudges the student's
body into alignment or demonstrates how a performance technique should
feel in fighting application. When I finally started to experience kung fu as
Master Jim intended, I discovered that my performative power was more
than I could have achieved on my own. My teacher had empowered me
with his own body-knowledge, taking my kung fu demonstrations to another level that elicited compliments from practitioners and observers alike
at Hong Luck's anniversary banquets. Consequently, I have come to understand body-experience lineage as an endowment that sustains the practice of
future generations. Even though Master Jim has departed from this world,
I can still feel him, adeptly guiding my kung fu when I practise. It is my sincere hope that this book will bring honour to him by helping to perpetuate
his legacy for the next generation.

Martial Sound and a Legacy of Musicking

The following ethnographic example will help show an important part of the
legacy that Master Jim wished to establish with regard to percussion beats.

For Hong Luck's fifty-fifth-anniversary banquet in 2016, the club's president tasked David with mounting a short drum show. Normally, Hong Luck's percussionists accompany lion dancing and kung fu demonstrations, only playing on their own to warm up the room. In this case, however, they were going to be on stage for a five-minute show. I volunteered to help, and the ensemble consisted of David on the drum, me on gong, and Bee on cymbals. David seized the opportunity to be creative, and he wanted to focus on using uncommon rhythms from Hong Luck's repertoire, as well as incorporating influences from other styles of lion dance drumming. As a group, we spent approximately one month piecing together the show, which we did in the weekly lion dance and advanced kung fu classes. In order to honour Master Jim, we included a small sample of his Taishanese walking beats. David also wanted to incorporate some different rhythms that he liked from the on-line videos of lion dance groups in Hong Kong, especially ones where the cymbalist(s) and gong player held a syncopated ostinato while the drummer improvised. Likewise, we borrowed ideas from videos of gong and drum ensembles in Malaysia and Singapore, where drum shows are becoming more popular. We even brought in some material that evoked West African drumming through the use of three-over-two polyrhythms. Everything was grafted onto Hong Luck's standard lion dance percussion beats, beginning and ending with the three-bows rhythm.

David's creative decisions were not without controversy, and some senior members raised concerns that these aesthetic choices were not traditional enough. For example, David wanted a section with a clave-esque timeline ostinato on the gong and cymbals that would anchor a semi-improvised drum solo. Master Jim was opposed, calling it categorically "incorrect" [mh dāk, 唔得]. On the surface, the problem seemed to be about traditional aesthetics: the percussion ensemble plays together and stops together, creating a continuously fulsome sonic texture. In standard kung fu and lion dance beats, the drummer is the leader, and so the other instrumentalists stop playing when there are significant rests in the drum part. In old-school Taishan lion beats, the integration is particularly tight and verges on monophony. Instead, David's solo involved many dramatic pauses where the gong and cymbal ostinato continued without him.

Master Jim was actually less concerned about what rhythms we played than he was with how we played them; he seemed not to care if we used new rhythms or old ones, as long as we played them in a way that musicked the appropriate sonic and choreomusical relationships. From his perspective, a continuous timeline supporting improvisation was not appropriate because it lacked togetherness. Rather than being a question of musical arrangement, the problem had to do with the meanings of the musicking, which Master Jim insisted were about being "together" [yāt chàih, 一齊]. Martial sound percussionists playing together are meant to auralize an esprit de corps, a spirit of cooperation, and a stance on unity, which does not leave room for independent drum solos. During rehearsals, Master Jim listened attentively and then offered feedback. Apart from the communal aspects of performance, he referred us back to how the emotional content of lion dance percussion is attached to intertextual choreomusical meanings—even when there is no choreography. When the drummer stops, not only should the metallophone players stop, but so should the lion dancers. Master Jim was concerned that the audience would be unable to feel embodied implications in the rhythms, which he suggested would then be "meaningless" [móuh yisī, 冇意思].

The musicking David chose was driven by musical concerns, rather than relationships between sound and movement, which showed his artistic stance on drumming and suggested a gong and drum ensemble may be able to play music after all. The actual performance at the anniversary banquet was successful, breaking new musical ground for the club and receiving a nice round of applause from the audience. As we descended from the stage, Master Jim commented to me, "néihdeih dōu hóyíh" [你哋都可以], meaning we had been alright or also acceptable, but his face showed that he was unimpressed. To be fair, David had been given the prerogative to do something different. A few weeks later, I apologized for our performance, and I tried to explain that David has his own drumming style. Master Jim replied that he was proud of David's talent, but he was still disappointed that the drum show had not adequately reflected Hong Luck's legacy of unity or his own lineage of Taishanese drumming. Nonetheless, our dearly departed master can rest assured that David is entirely ready, willing, and able to preserve, transmit, perform, and promote traditional gong and drum beats—despite having jumped at the chance to play a bit of music.

Implications of Martial Sound for Research and Practice

Martial sound is a way we can listen to music as martial arts and a way that martial arts can be heard as musicking. By being attentive to the total soundscape of martial arts, I suggest that scholars and practitioners alike can enhance their understanding of teaching, learning, practising, performing, and even fighting. In this book I have provided extensive ethnographic examples of how martial sound works in a Chinese Canadian kung fu club. Now I distil the specifics into a more general concept, with broader application. The conceptual distillate falls into three main areas where martial sound is at work: social, personal, and, of course, martial. My disciplinary orientation is musical, and so there are bound to be overlaps with the meanings and uses of music more generally. What I want to highlight are the martial qualities that sound and music can have, which, notwithstanding work like that of Martin Daughtry (2015), are under-represented in scholarly discourse.

On a social level, martial sound organizes, motivates, connects, builds, and teaches. Whether in an instructor's measured counting to keep beginners in time during practice or in musical rhythms that set the timing for performers, players, dancers, and competitors, martial sound is organizing. Martial sound is motivating and provides energy to participants that can push them to higher levels of focus and exertion. In connecting groups of people through sound, it allows practitioners and audiences to hear the movement of others whom they cannot see. Through connections established in practice and performance, martial sound works at building community. Finally, martial sound is useful for teaching, as when the rhythm of combat can be made explicit for students. The ability to form sonic and kinetic relationships in time is common to other types of musicking (Small 1998; Turino 2008), but it is all too easy to overlook in the context of fighting arts. Rather than treating it as a supplement to the main social and combative functions, I reposition martial sound at the centre of the action.

On a personal level, martial sound constructs, contests, negotiates, and performs, as well as assists learning and leads to being. As embodied practices, martial arts are exceptionally demanding because of their engagement with the spectre of violence—real or imagined. Through the practice of hand combat, people are radically reconstructing their identities to become warriors, and they cannot do so quietly. In many martial arts, a cultural, ethnic, or national element is also an important part of identity construction, and sonic aspects are central to performing in a coherent way. Nonetheless, practitioners are typically contesting and negotiating the meanings of their identities in an active manner, deploying martial sound to counter, influence, or reinforce the perceptions of others. As a tool for learning, martial sound provides a sensorial guide that complements and enhances linguistic explanations or embodied demonstrations. Lastly, engaging with the soundscape of hand combat is integral to martial being-in-the-world, and practitioners actualize their lived realities multi-modally to achieve the most immersive effect. Martial arts studies scholars are well aware of identity work in hand combat (Frank 2006; Facal 2017), but I am emphasizing the importance of sound to that work, lest it be overlooked.

On a martial level, sound and music empower, intimidate, dominate, claim, and resist, while also contributing to strategy. Military music has long been valued for intimidating an enemy at a distance, announcing the presence, strength, and organization of trained fighters. Similarly, battle cries and primal screams are used to strike terror into the hearts of adversaries. At high volume, martial sound of all varieties is used for dominating an encounter by drowning out the opposition. In non-combative situations, extending the reach of heroic displays through martial sound enhances the claiming of space during parades. Likewise, demonstrations and protests deploy martial sound through music, chants, claps, whistles, and so on as a way of sonically resisting various forms of social, political, and economic oppression by showing support, strength, and unity in opposition. Strategically, hearing and using martial sound opens up the rhythm of combat to be recognized, analysed, manipulated, and controlled for devastating effect.

In conclusion, I would like to offer a few provocations. This book has demonstrated a method of listening to martial arts, including the musicking of combat, ritual, and performance. It is my hope that this research will help scholars, practitioners, and audiences alike to attune their senses to a different way of hearing sound and music in hand combat. More broadly, listening to human activity for its sonic and rhythmic qualities presents opportunities for understanding the world around us more deeply, as well as for hearing things that we had not previously noticed. Musicking is part of many types of meaningful action in which it is not the focus, but that does not mean it is dispensable. Unfortunately, the integral sonic aspects of some cultural expressions may go unremarked when they are not culturally constructed as "music"—despite clearly being musicking. Moreover, sound is all around us, but a verbal and visual bias can obscure important auditory information. Whether in the timing of a joke's punch line, the ping of a bat's sweet spot hitting a ball, the sonic texture of ritual practices, or the rhythm patterns of a basketball player dribbling their way down the court, there is a whole world of sound waiting to be discovered.

Works Cited

al Faruqi, Lois Ibsen. 1978. "Accentuation in Qur'ānic Chant: A Study in Musical Tawāzun." *Yearbook of the International Folk Music Council* 10: 53–68.

al Faruqi, Lois Ibsen. 1985. "Music, Musicians and Muslim Law." *Asian Music* 17(1): 3–36.

Anderson, Benedict R. 2006 (1983). *Imagined Communities: Reflections on the Origin and Spread of Nationalism*, revised edition. London: Verso.

Bakan, Michael. 1999. *Music of Death and New Creation: Experiences in the World of Balinese Gamelan Beleganjur*. Chicago: University of Chicago Press.

Barz, Gregory, and Timothy J. Cooley, eds. 2008 [1997]. *Shadows in the Field: New Perspectives for Fieldwork in Ethnomusicology*, second edition. New York: Oxford University Press.

Benson, Bruce. 2003. *The Improvisation of Musical Dialogue: A Phenomenology of Music*. Cambridge: Cambridge University Press.

Berger, Harris M. 2008 [1997]. "Phenomenology and the Ethnography of Popular Music: Ethnomusicology at the Juncture of Cultural Studies and Folklore." In *Shadows in the Field: New Perspectives for Fieldwork in Ethnomusicology*, second edition, ed. Gregory F. Barz and Timothy J. Cooley, 62–75. New York: Oxford University Press.

Berger, Harris M. 2009. *Stance: Ideas About Emotion, Style, and Meaning in the Study of Expressive Culture*. Middletown, CT: Wesleyan University Press.

Bithell, Caroline. 2003. "A Man's Game? Engendered Song and the Changing Dynamic of Musical Activity in Corsica." In *Music and Gender: Perspectives from the Mediterranean*, ed. Tullia Magrini, 33–66. Chicago: University of Chicago Press.

Blacking, John. 1973. *How Musical Is Man?* Seattle: University of Washington Press.

Blue, Stanley. 2014. "Shaping the Rhythms of Mixed Martial Arts Practice." In *Fighting: Intellectualising Combat Sports*, ed. Keith Gilbert, 117–124. Champaign, IL: Common Ground Publishing.

Bolelli, Danielle. 2003. *On the Warrior's Path: Philosophy, Fighting, and Martial Arts Mythology*. Berkeley, CA: Frog Books.

Boretz, Avron. 2011. *Gods, Ghosts, and Gangsters: Ritual Violence, Martial Arts, and Masculinity on the Margins of Chinese Society*. Honolulu: University of Hawai'i Press.

Bourdieu, Pierre. 1977 [1972]. *Outline of a Theory of Practice*. Trans. Richard Nice. New York: Cambridge University Press.

Bourdieu, Pierre. 1990 [1980]. *The Logic of Practice*. Trans. Richard Nice. Stanford, CA: Stanford University Press.

Bowman, Paul. 2013. *Beyond Bruce Lee: Chasing the Dragon Through Film, Philosophy and Popular Culture*. New York: Wallflower Press.

Bowman, Paul. 2015. *Martial Arts Studies: Disrupting Disciplinary Boundaries*. London: Rowman and Littlefield.

Bowman, Paul. 2016. "The Definition of Martial Arts Studies." *Martial Arts Studies* 3: 6–23.

Brown, David. 2014. "Body-experience Lineages in Martial Art Cultures." In *Fighting: Intellectualising Combat Sports*, ed. Keith Gilbert, 67–77. Champaign, IL: Common Ground Publishing.

Butler, Judith. 1988. "Performative Acts and Gender Constitution: An Essay in Phenomenology and Feminist Theory." *Theatre Journal* 40(4): 519–531.

Campbell, Patricia Shehan, and Kuo-Huang Han. 1996. *The Lion's Roar: Chinese Percussion Ensembles*, second edition. Danbury, CT: World Music Press.

Ceccagno, Antonella. 2006. "Gender in Chinese and New Writing Technologies." In *Gender, Language and New Literacy*, ed. Eva-Maria Thüne, Simona Leonardi, and Carla Bazzanella, 213–230. London: Continuum.

Chakrabarty, Dipesh. 2000. *Provincializing Europe: Postcolonial Thought and Historical Difference*. Princeton, NJ: Princeton University Press.

Chan, Arlene. 2011. *The Chinese in Toronto from 1878: From Outside to Inside the Circle*. Toronto, ON: Dundern Press.

Chan, Mei Hsiu. 2001. "Transdisciplinary Multicultural Dance Education: Teaching Chinese American Students Chinese Culture through Lion Dancing." PhD diss., Texas Women's University.

Chernoff, John Miller. 1979. *African Rhythm and African Sensibility: Aesthetics and Social Action in African Musical Idioms*. Chicago: Chicago University Press.

Chou, Chiener. 2002. "Learning Processes in the *Nanguan* Music of Taiwan." *British Journal of Ethnomusicology* 11(2): 81–124.

Clayton, Martin, Rebecca Sager, and Udo Will. 2004. "In Time with the Music: The Concept of Entrainment and its Significance for Ethnomusicology." *European Meetings in Ethnomusicology* 11: 3–75.

Cleary, Thomas, trans. 2003. *The Art of War: Complete Texts and Commentary*. Boston: Shambhala Publications.

Cooley, Timothy J. 2006. "Folk Festival as Modern Ritual in the Polish Tatra Mountains." In *Ethnomusicology: A Contemporary Reader*, ed. Jennifer Post, 67–84. New York: Routledge.

Cornford, Francis MacDonald, trans. 1972. *The Republic of Plato*. New York: Oxford University Press.

Cowan, Jane K. 1990. *Dance and the Body Politic in Northern Greece*. Princeton, NJ: Princeton University Press.

Csordas, Thomas J. 1990. "Embodiment as a Paradigm for Anthropology." *Ethos* 18(1): 5–47.

Daughtry, J. Martin. 2015. *Listening to War: Sound, Music, Trauma, and Survival in Wartime Iraq*. New York: Oxford University Press.

DeKorne, John C. 1934. "Sun Yat-Sen and the Secret Societies." *Pacific Affairs* 17(4): 425–433.

Delamont, Sara, and Neil Stephens. 2008. "Up on the Roof: The Embodied Habitus of Diasporic *Capoeira*." *Cultural Sociology* 2(1): 57–74.

Diaz, Juan Diego. 2017. "Between Repetition and Variation: A Musical Performance of *Malícia* in Capoeira." *Ethnomusicology Forum* 26(1): 46–68.

Dong, Xuan. 2016. "Being Tough and Belonging: Technologies of Masculinity among Martial Arts Students in China." *The Asia Pacific Journal of Anthropology* 17(1): 34–49.

Donohue, John. 2000. "Sound and Fury: Auditory Elements in Martial Ritual." *Journal of the Asian Martial Arts* 9(4): 12–20.

Downey, Greg. 2002. "Listening to Capoeira: Phenomenology, Embodiment, and the Materiality of Music." *Ethnomusicology* 46(3): 487–509.

Downey, Greg. 2005. *Learning Capoeira: Lessons in Cunning from an Afro-Brazilian Art*. New York: Oxford University Press.

Downey, Greg, Monica Dalidowicz, and Paul H. Mason. 2014. "Apprenticeship as Method: Embodied Learning in Ethnographic Practice." *Qualitative Research* 15(2): 183–200.

Duara, Prasenjit. 1988. "Superscribing Symbols: The Myth of Guandi, Chinese God of War." *The Journal of Asian Studies* 47(4): 778–795.

Echard, William. 1999. "An Analysis of Neil Young's 'Powderfinger' Based on Mark Johnson's Image Schemata." *Popular Music* 18(1): 133–144.

Facal, Gabriel. 2017. "Trans-regional Continuities of Fighting Techniques in Martial Ritual Initiations of the Malay World." *Martial Arts Studies* 4: 46–69.

Farrer, D. S. 2009. *Shadows of the Prophet: Martial Arts and Sufi Mysticism*. Muslims in Global Society 2. Dordrecht, NL: Springer.

Farrer, D. S. 2011. "Coffee-Shop Gods: Chinese Martial Arts of the Singapore Diaspora." In *Martial Arts as Embodied Knowledge: Asian Traditions in a Transnational World*, ed. D. S. Farrer and John Whalen-Bridge, 4035–4799. Kindle edition. Albany, NY: SUNY Press.

Farrer, D. S. 2015. "Efficacy and Entertainment in Martial Arts Studies: Anthropological Perspectives." *Martial Arts Studies* 1: 34–45.

Feld, Steven. 1990. *Sound and Sentiment: Birds, Weeping, Poetics, and Song in Kaluli Expression*, second edition. Philadelphia, PA: University of Pennsylvania Press.

Feltham, Heleanor B. 2009. "Everybody Was Kung-Fu Fighting: The Lion Dance and Chinese National Identity in the 19th and 20th Centuries." In *Asian Material Culture*, ed. Marianne Hulbosch, Elizabeth Bedford, and Martha Chaiklin, 103–140. Amsterdam: Amsterdam University Press.

Fogelsanger, Allen, and Kathleya Afanador. 2006. "Parameters of Perception: Vision, Audition, and Twentieth-Century Music and Dance." Paper presented in the Congress on Research in Dance, Tempe, Arizona, 2–5 November.

Frank, Adam D. 2006. *Taijiquan and the Search for the Little Old Chinese Man: Understanding Identity through the Martial Arts*. New York: Palgrave MacMillan.

Freudenthal, Hans. 1991. *Revisiting Mathematics Education: China Lectures*. Dordrecht, NL: Kluwer Academic Publishers.

Friedson, Steven. 1996. *Dancing Prophets: Musical Experiences in Tumbuka Healing*. Chicago: University of Chicago Press.

Frith, Simon. 1996. *Performing Rites: On the Value of Popular Music*. Cambridge, MA: Harvard University Press.

Gawlikowski, Krzysztof. 1987. "The Concept of Two Fundamental Social Principles: Wen 文 and Wu 武 in Chinese Classical Thought (Part I)." *Annali di Istituto Italiano per l'Africa e l'Oriente* 47: 397–433.

Gawlikowski, Krzysztof. 1988. "The Concept of Two Fundamental Social Principles: Wen 文 and Wu 武 in Chinese Classical Thought (Part II)." *Annali di Istituto Italiano per l'Africa e l'Oriente* 48(1): 35–64.

Geertz, Clifford. 1973. *The Interpretation of Cultures: Selected Essays*. New York: Basic Books.

Geertz, Clifford. 1980. "Blurred Genres: The Refiguration of Social Thought." *The American Scholar* 49(2): 165–179.

Geertz, Clifford. 1983. *Local Knowledge: Further Essays in Interpretive Anthropology*. New York: Basic Books.

Geertz, Clifford. 1998. "Deep Hanging Out." *New York Review of Books* 45(16): 69–72.

Gillborn, D. 2006. "Rethinking White Supremacy: Who Counts in 'WhiteWorld.'" *Ethnicities* 6(3): 318–340.

Goodman, Steve. 2010. *Sonic Warfare: Sound, Affect, and the Ecology of Fear*. Cambridge, MA: The MIT Press.

Green, Thomas A. 2001. "Introduction." In *Martial Arts of the World: An Encyclopedia. Volume One: A–Q*, ed. Thomas Green, xv–xviii. Santa Barbara, CA: ABC Clio.

Green, Thomas A. 2003. "Sense in Nonsense: The Role of Folk History in the Martial Arts." In *Martial Arts in the Modern World*, ed. Thomas A. Green and Joseph R. Svinth, 1–11. Westport, CT: Praeger.

Green, Thomas A., and Joseph R. Svinth, eds. 2003. *Martial Arts in the Modern World*. Westport, CT: Praeger.

Hahn, Tomie. 2007. *Sensational Knowledge: Embodying Culture Through Japanese Dance*. Middleton, CT: Wesleyan University Press.

Harrell, Steven. 1977. "Modes of Belief in Chinese Folk Religion." *Journal for the Scientific Study of Religion* 16(1): 55–65.

Heidegger, Martin. 1977 [1950]. "Origin of the Work of Art." In *Basic Writings*, ed. David Farrell Krell, 149–187. San Francisco, CA: Harper.

Henning, Stanley E. 1981. "The Chinese Martial Arts in Historical Perspective." *Society for Military History* 45(4): 173–179.

Henning, Stanley E. 1984. "Ignorance, Legend and Taijiquan." *Journal of the Chen Style Taijiquan Research Association of Hawaii* 2(3): 1–7.

Henning, Stanley E. 1999. "Academia Encounters the Chinese Martial Arts." *China Review International* 6(2): 319–332.

Henning, Stanley E. 2006. "China's New Wave of Martial Studies Scholars." *Journal of Asian Martial Arts* 15(2): 8–21.

Hobsbawm, Eric, and Terence Ranger, eds. 1983. *The Invention of Tradition*. Cambridge: University of Cambridge Press.

Hodgins, Paul. 1992. *Music, Movement, and Metaphor: Relationships Between Score and Choreography in Twentieth-century Dance*. New York: Edwin Mellin Press.

Holcombe, Charles. 2002. "Theatre of Combat: A Critical Look at the Chinese Martial Arts." In *Combat, Ritual, and Performance: Anthropology of the Martial Arts*, ed. David E. Jones, 153–173. Westport, CT: Praeger Publishers.

Hood, Mantle. 1960. "The Challenge of 'Bi-Musicality.'" *Ethnomusicology* 4(2): 55–59.

Hsu, Adam. 1998. *The Sword Polisher's Record: The Way of Kung Fu*. Boston: Tuttle Publishing.

Hu, William C. C. 1995. *Chinese Lion Dance Explained*. San Francisco, CA: Ars Ceramica.

Husserl, Edmund. 1962 [1913]. *Ideas: General Introduction to Pure Phenomenology*. Trans. W. R. Boyce Gibson. New York: Collier Books.

Husserl, Edmund. 1964 [1928]. *Phenomenology of Internal Time Consciousness*. Trans. James S. Churchill. Bloomington, IL: Indiana University Press.

Husserl, Edmund. 1970 [1900]. *Logical Investigations: Volume 1*. Trans. J. N. Findlay. London: Routledge & Kegan Paul.

Ihde, Don. 2007 [1976]. *Listening and Voice: A Phenomenology of Sound*. Athens: Ohio University Press.

Johnson, Henry. 2005. "Dancing with Lions: (Per)forming Chinese Cultural Identity at a New Zealand Secondary School." *New Zealand Journal of Asian Studies* 7(2): 171–186.

Johnson, Mark. 1987. *The Body in the Mind: The Bodily Basis of Meaning, Imagination, and Reason*. Chicago: University of Chicago Press.

Johnson, Mark. 1997/1998. "Embodied Musical Meaning." *Theory and Practice* 22/23: 95–102.

Jones, David E., ed. 2002a. *Combat, Ritual, and Performance: Anthropology of the Martial Arts*. Westport, CT: Praeger Publishers.

Jones, David E. 2002b. "Towards a Definition of the Martial Arts." In *Combat, Ritual, and Performance: Anthropology of the Martial Arts*, ed. David E. Jones, xi–xv. Westport, CT: Praeger.

Jones, Stephen. 1995. *Folk Music of China: Living Instrumental Traditions*. New York: Oxford University Press.

Jones, Stephen. 1996. "Source and Stream: Early Music and Living Traditions in China." *Early Music* 24(3): 374–378.

Jordan, Stephanie. 2011. "Choreomusical Conversations: Facing a Double Challenge." *Dance Research Journal* 43(1): 43–64.

Judkins, Benjamin N. 2014. "Inventing Kung Fu." *JOMEC Journal* 5: 1–23.

Judkins, Benjamin N. 2016. "The Seven Forms of Lightsaber Combat: Hyper-reality and the Invention of the Martial Arts." *Martial Arts Studies* 2: 6–22.

Judkins, Benjamin N., and Jon Nielson. 2015. *The Creation of Wing Chun: A Social History of the Southern Chinese Martial Arts*. Albany, NY: SUNY Press.

Kaeppler, Adrienne L. 2001. "Ethnochoreology." *Grove Music Online*. Accessed August 8, 2018. https://doi.org/10.1093/gmo/9781561592630.article.40752.

Kapleau, Philip, ed. 1965. *The Three Pillars of Zen: Teaching Practice Enlightenment*. Boston: Beacon Press.

Kastin, David. 1985. "Lee Konitz: Back to Basics." *Downbeat* December: 54–56.

Keil, Charles. 1987. "Participatory Discrepancies and the Power of Music." *Cultural Anthropology* 2(3): 275–283.

Kennedy, Brian, and Elizabeth Guo. 2005. *Chinese Martial Arts Training Manuals: A Historical Survey*. Berkeley, CA: Blue Snake Books.

Kenny, Ailbhe. 2016. *Communities of Musical Practice*. New York: Routledge.

Kerman, Joseph. 1985. *Contemplating Music: Challenges to Musicology*. Cambridge, MA: Harvard University Press.

Keulemans, Paize. 2014. *Sounds Rising from the Paper: Nineteenth-Century Martial Arts Fiction and the Chinese Acoustic Imagination.* Cambridge, MA: Harvard University Press.

Kim, Han-Gu. 1975. "An Anthropological Perspective on the Lion Dance." *Korea Journal* 15(25): 29–37.

Kippen, James. 2008 [1997]. "Working with the Masters." In *Shadows in the Field: New Perspectives for Fieldwork in Ethnomusicology,* second edition, ed. Gregory Barz and Timothy J. Cooley, 125–140. New York: Oxford University Press.

Klens-Bigman. 2002. "Towards a Theory of Martial Arts as Performance Art." In *Combat, Ritual, and Performance: Anthropology of the Martial Arts,* ed. David E. Jones, 1–10. Westport, CT: Praeger.

Klens-Bigman. 2007. "Yet More Towards a Theory of Martial Arts as Performing Art." *InYo: Journal of Alternative Perspectives* 7(December): 1–6.

Knoblock, John, and Jeffrey Riegel, trans. 2000. *The Annals of Lü Buwei* [呂氏春秋]. Stanford, CA: Stanford University Press.

Koskoff, Ellen, ed. 1987. *Women and Music in Cross-cultural Perspective.* Chicago: University of Illinois Press.

Kozub, Francis M., and Mary L. Kozub. 2004. "Teaching Combative Sports Through Tactics." *Journal of Physical Education Recreation and Dance* 75(8): 16–21.

Lai, David Chuenyan. 2011. *A Brief Chronology of Chinese Canadian History: From Segregation to Integration.* Burnaby, BC: Simon Fraser University, David See-Chai Lam Centre for International Communication.

Lai, David Chuenyan, and Jack Leong. 2012. *Toronto Chinatowns 1878–2012.* Burnaby, BC: Simon Fraser University, David See-Chai Lam Centre for International Communication.

Lave, Jean, and Etienne Wenger. 1991. *Situated Learning: Legitimate Peripheral Participation.* Cambridge: Cambridge University Press.

Lee, Aaron. n.d. "A Visit to Sifu Lok So: The Tao Style." Location/publisher unknown. (magazine article on the wall of the Hong Luck Kung Fu Club about Do Pi, featuring an interview with the founder's top disciple).

Lee, Bruce. 1975. *Tao of Jeet Kune Do.* Santa Clarita, CA: Ohara.

Lee, Koon-Hung. 1983. *Choy Lay Fut Kung Fu: The Dynamic Art of Fighting.* Hong Kong: Lee Koon-Hung Publishing Company.

Lewis, J. Lowell. 1992. *Ring of Liberation: Deceptive Discourse in Brazilian Capoeira.* Chicago: University of Chicago Press.

Li, Mu. 2017. "Performing Chineseness: The Lion Dance in Newfoundland." *Asian Ethnology* 76(2): 289–317.

Li, Peter. 1998. *The Chinese in Canada,* second edition. Don Mills, ON: Oxford University Press.

Li, Zeqin, and Guozhi Liu, eds. 1985. *A Collection of Folk 'Lantern' Performances* [李则琴 刘国治主编]. Nanchang: Jiangxi Xinhua Printing House.

Liang, Jufa. 2008. *Southern Lion* [南狮]. China: International Book Publishing.

Lin, Yatin. 2010. "Choreographing a Flexible Taiwan: Cloud Gate Dance Theatre and Taiwan's Changing Identity." In *The Routledge Dance Studies Reader,* second edition, ed. Alexandra Carter and Janet O'Shea, 225–260. New York: Routledge.

Liu, Chang-lin. 2011. "On Artistic Characteristics of Nanhai Lion Drum-music in Foshan" [南海醒狮鼓乐"桩狮" 鼓点艺术特征分析]. *Journal of Xinghai Conservatory of Music* 2: 45–50.

Liu, Jing, and Han-qiao Yu. 2007. "On Modernization Development of Lion Dance and Dragon Dance as National Traditional Sports in View of Culture Structure" [从文化结构看民族传统体育舞龙舞狮运动的现代化发展]. *Journal of Beijing Sport University* 2007(7): 889–891.

Liu, Wanyu. 1981. "The Chinese Lion Dance." MFA thesis, York University.

Lorge, Peter. 2012. *Chinese Martial Arts: From Antiquity to the 21st Century.* New York: Cambridge University Press.

Louie, Kam. 2002. *Theorising Chinese Masculinity: Society and Gender in China*. Cambridge: Cambridge University Press.

Ma, Mingda. 2003. *Seeking the Facts in Martial Studies* [武學探真]. 2 vols. Taibei: Yi Wen Press.

Martinez, Alejandra. 2014. "No Longer a Girl: My Female Experience in the Masculine Field of Martial Arts." *International Review of Qualitative Research* 7(4): 442–452.

Mason, Paul H. 2012. "Music, Dance and the Total Art Work: Choreomusicology in Theory and Practice." *Research in Dance Education* 13(1): 5–24.

Mason, Paul H. 2014. "Tapping the Plate or Hitting the Bottle: Sound and Movement in Self-accompanied and Musician-accompanied Dance." *Ethnomusicology Forum* 23(2): 208–228.

Mason, Paul H. 2016a. "Silek Minang in West Sumatra, Indonesia." In *The Fighting Art of Pencak Silat and its Music: From Southeast Asian Village to Global Movement*, ed. Uwe Paetzold and Paul H. Mason, 205–234. Leiden, NL: Koninklijke Brill NV.

Mason, Paul H. 2016b. "Pencak Silat Seni in West Java, Indonesia." In *The Fighting Art of Pencak Silat and its Music: From Southeast Asian Village to Global Movement*, ed. Uwe Paetzold and Paul H. Mason, 235–264. Leiden, NL: Koninklijke Brill NV.

Mason, Paul H. 2016c. "Fight-dancing and the Festival: Tabuik in Parjaman, Indonesia, and Iemanjá in Salvador da Bahia, Brazil." *Martial Arts Studies Journal* 2: 71–90.

Mason, Paul H. 2017. "Combat-dancing, Cultural Transmission and Choreomusicology: The Globalization of Embodied Repertoires of Sound and Movement." In *The Routledge Companion to Embodied Music Interaction*; ed. Micheline Lesaffre, Pieter-Jan Maes, and Marc Leman; 223–231. New York: Routledge.

Mauss, Marcel. 1934. "Les techniques du corps." *Journal de Psychologie* 32(3–4): 5–23.

May, Reinhard. 1996 [1989]. *Heidegger's Hidden Sources: East Asian Influences on His Work*. Trans. Graham Parkes. New York: Routledge.

Merleau-Ponty, Maurice. 2002 [1942]. *Phenomenology of Perception*. Trans. Colin Smith. New York: Routledge.

McClary, Susan. 1994. "Paradigm Dissonances: Music Theory, Cultural Studies, Feminist Criticism." *Perspectives of New Music* 32(1): 68–85.

McGuire, Colin. 2010. "Rhythm Skills Development in Chinese Martial Arts." *The International Journal of Sport and Society* 1(3): 209–218.

McGuire, Colin. 2015. "The Rhythm of Combat: Understanding the Role of Music in Performances of Traditional Chinese Martial Arts and Lion Dance." *MUSICultures* 42(1): 1–23.

McGuire, Colin. 2018. "Unisonance in Kung Fu Film Music, or the Wong Fei-hung Theme Song as a Cantonese Transnational Anthem." *Ethnomusicology Forum* 27(1): 48–67.

McGuire, Colin. 2019 "Timing in Bruce Lee's Writings as Inspiration for Listening Musically to Hand Combat and Martial Arts Performance." *Martial Arts Studies* 8: 73–83.

McNeil, William H. 1995. *Keeping Together in Time: Dance and Drill in Human History*. Cambridge, MA: Harvard University Press.

Merriam, Alan P. 1964. *The Anthropology of Music*. Evanston, IL: Northwestern University Press.

Miyamoto, Musashi. 1982. *The Book of Five Rings*. Trans. Nihon Services Corporation. New York: Bantam. Original edition, Japan: letter to Terao Magonojo, 1645.

Monson, Ingrid. 1999. "Riffs, Repetition, and Theories of Globalization." *Ethnomusicology* 43(1): 31–65.

Morris, Andrew. 2004. *Marrow of the Nations: A History of Sport and Physical Culture in Republican China*. Berkeley, CA: University of California Press.

Murray, Dian H., and Baoqi Qin. 1994. *The Origins of the Tiandihui: The Chinese Triads in Legend and History*. Stanford, CA: Stanford University Press.

Nattiez, Jean-Jacques. 1999. "Inuit Throat-Games and Siberian Throat Singing: A Comparative, Historical, and Semiological Approach." *Ethnomusicology* 43(3): 399–418.

Ness, Sally Ann. 1992. *Body, Movement, and Culture: Kineasthetic and Visual Symbolism in a Philippine Community*. Philadelphia, PA: University of Pennsylvania Press.

Nettl, Bruno. 2005 [1983]. *The Study of Ethnomusicology: Thirty-One Issues and Concepts.* New Edition. Urbana and Chicago: University of Illinois Press.

Nye, Joseph S. Jr. 1990. "Soft Power." *Foreign Policy* 80: 153–171.

Ownby, David. 1995. "The Heaven and Earth Society as Popular Religion." *The Journal of Asian Studies* 54(4): 1023–1046.

Paetzold, Uwe U., and Paul H. Mason, eds. 2016. *The Fighting Art of Pencak Silat and Its Music: From Southeast Asian Village to Global Movement.* Leiden, NL: Koninklijke Brill NV.

Parkes, Graham, ed. 1987. *Heidegger and Asian Thought.* Honolulu: University of Hawai'i Press.

Peirce, Charles. 1985 (1903). "Logic as Semiotic: The Theory of Signs." In *Semiotics: An Introductory Anthology*, ed. Robert Innis, 4–23. Bloomington: University of Indiana Press.

Phillips, Scott Park. 2016. *Possible Origins: A Cultural History of Chinese Martial Arts, Theatre, and Religion.* N.P.: Angry Baby Books.

Phillips-Silver, Jessica, C. Athena Aktipis, and Gregory A. Bryant. 2010. "The Ecology of Entrainment: Foundations of Coordinated Rhythmic Movement." *Music Perception: An Interdisciplinary Journal* 28(10): 3–14.

Qureshi, Regula Burckhardt. 1986. *Sufi Music of India and Pakistan: Sound Context, and Meaning in Qawwali.* Cambridge: Cambridge University Press.

Rahaim, Matthew. 2012. *Musicking Bodies: Gesture and Voice in Hindustani Music.* Middletown, CT: Wesleyan University Press.

Raulin, Anne. 1991. "The Aesthetic and Sacred Dimension of Urban Ecology: Paris' Little Asia." Trans. Jeanne Brody. *Archives de sciences socials des religions* 36(73): 35–49.

Reybrouck, Mark. 2001 "Musical Imagery between Sensory Processing and Ideomotor Simulation." In *Musical Imagery*, ed. R. I. Godøy and H. Jörgensen, 117–132. Lisse, NL: Swets and Zeitlinger.

Rice, Timothy. 1994. *May it Fill Your Soul: Experiencing Bulgarian Folk Music.* Chicago: University of Chicago Press.

Rice, Timothy. 2003. "The Ethnomusicology of Learning and Teaching." *College Music Symposium* 43: 65–85.

Rice, Timothy. 2008 [1997]. "Toward a Mediation of Field Methods and Field Experience in Ethnomusicology." In *Shadows in the Field: New Perspectives for Fieldwork in Ethnomusicology*, second edition, ed. Gregory F. Barz and Timothy J. Cooley, 42–61. New York: Oxford University Press.

Rice, Timothy. 2010. "Ethnomusicological Theory." *Yearbook for Traditional Music* 42: 100–134.

Ricoeur, Paul. 1984. "The Model of the Text: Meaningful Action Considered as a Text." *Social Research* 51(1/2): 185–218.

Rollefson, J. Griffith. 2017. "Hip Hop as Martial Art: Towards a Political Economy of Violence in Rap Music." In *The Oxford Handbook of Hip Hop Studies*, ed. Justin Burton and Jason Oakes. New York: Oxford University Press. https://doi.org/10.1093/oxfordhb/9780190281090.013.11

Sager, Rebecca. 2012. "Transcendence through Aesthetic Experience: Divining a Common Wellspring under Conflicting Caribbean and African American Religious Value Systems." *Black Music Research Journal* 32(1): 27–67.

Schafer, R. Murray. 1993. *The Soundscape: Our Sonic Environment and the Tuning of the World.* Rochester, VT: Destiny Books.

Schechner, Richard. 1974. "From Ritual to Theatre and Back: The Structure/Process of the Efficacy-Entertainment Dyad." *Educational Theatre Journal* 26(4): 455–481.

Schechner, Richard. 1993. *The Future of Ritual: Writings on Culture and Performance.* New York: Routledge.

Schieffelin, Edward. 1985. "Performance and the Cultural Construction of Reality." *American Ethnologist* 12(4): 707–724.

Scott, David. 2008. *China and the International System, 1840–1949: Power, Presence, and Perceptions in a Century of Humiliation.* Albany: State University of New York Press.

Seeger, Charles. 1958. "Prescriptive and Descriptive Music-Writing." *The Musical Quarterly* 44(2): 184–195.

Shahar, Meir. 2008. *The Shaolin Monastery: History, Religion, and the Chinese Martial Arts.* Honolulu: University of Hawai'i Press.

Slovenz, Madeline Anita. 1987. "'The Year is a Wild Animal': Lion Dancing in Chinatown." *The Drama Review* 31(3): 74–102.

Slovenz-Low, Madeline. 1994. "Lions in the Streets: A Performance Ethnography of Cantonese Lion Dancing in New York City's Chinatown." PhD diss., New York University.

Small, Christopher. 1998. *Musicking: The Meanings of Performing and Listening.* Middletown, CT: Wesleyan University Press.

Smart, Josephine. 2012. "Dancing with the Dragon: Canadian Investment in China and Chinese Investment in Canada." SPP Research Papers 5(27): 1–20.

Spatz, Ben. 2015 *What a Body Can Do: Technique as Knowledge, Practice as Research.* New York: Routledge.

Spencer, Dale. 2009. "Habit(us), Body Techniques and Body Callusing: An Ethnography of Mixed Martial Arts." *Body and Society* 15(4): 119–143.

Spencer, Dale, and Raúl Sánchez García, eds. 2013. *Fighting Scholars: Habitus and Ethnographies of Martial Arts and Combat Sports.* New York: Anthem Press.

Spivak, Gayatri Chakravorty. 1988. "Subaltern Studies: Deconstructing Historiography." In *Selected Subaltern Studies*, ed. Ranajit Guha and Gayatri Chakravorty Spivak, 3–32. Oxford: Oxford University Press.

Sterne, Jonathan. 2012. "Sonic Imaginations." In *The Sound Studies Reader*, ed. Jonathan Sterne, 1–17. New York: Routledge.

Stock, Jonathan P. J. 2002. "Learning 'Huju' in Shanghai, 1900–1950: Apprenticeship and the Acquisition of Expertise in a Chinese Local Opera Tradition." *Asian Music* 33(2): 1–42.

Stock, Jonathan P. J. 2004. "Documenting the Musical Event: Observation, Participation, Representation." In *Empirical Musicology: Aims, Methods, and Prospects*, ed. Eric Clarke and Nicholas Cooke, 15–34. New York: Oxford University Press.

Stock, Jonathan, and Chiener Chou. 2008 (1997). "Fieldwork at Home." In *Shadows in the Field: New Perspectives for Fieldwork in Ethnomusicology*, second edition, ed. Gregory Barz and Timothy J. Cooley, 108–124. New York: Oxford University Press.

Stone, Ruth. 1982. *Let the Inside be Sweet: The Interpretation of Music Event Among the Kpelle of Liberia.* Bloomington: University of Indiana Press.

Sugarman, Jane C. 1989. "The Nightingale and the Partridge: Singing and Gender among Prespa Albanians." *Ethmomusicology* 33(2): 191–215.

ter Haar, Barend J. 2000. *Ritual and Mythology of the Chinese Triads: Creating and Identity.* Boston: Brill Academic Publishers.

Thrasher, Alan R. 2008. *Sizhu Instrumental Music of South China: Ethos, Theory and Practice.* Leiden, NL: Koninklijke Brill NV.

Thompson, Richard H. 1989. *Toronto's Chinatown: The Changing Social Organization of an Ethnic Community.* New York: AMS Press.

Titon, Jeff Todd. 1988. *Powerhouse for God: Speech, Chant, and Song in an Appalachian Baptist Church.* Austin, TX: University of Texas Press.

Titon, Jeff Todd. 2008 [1997]. "Knowing Fieldwork." In *Shadows in the Field: New Perspectives for Fieldwork in Ethnomusicology*, second edition, ed. Gregory F. Barz and Timothy J. Cooley, 25–41. New York: Oxford University Press.

Torp, Jörgen. 2013. "Musical Movement: Towards a Common Term for Music and Dance." *Yearbook for Traditional Music* 45: 231–249.

Turino, Thomas. 2000. *Nationalists, Cosmopolitans, and Popular Music in Zimbabwe.* Chicago: University of Chicago Press.

Turino, Thomas. 2008. *Music as Social Life: The Politics of Participation.* Chicago: University of Chicago Press.

Turino, Thomas. 2014. "Peircean Thought as Core Theory for a Phenomenological Ethnomusicology." *Ethnomusicology* 58(2): 185–221

Turner, Victor. 1973. "Symbols in African Rituals." *Science* 179(4078): 1100–1105.

Turner, Victor. 1975. "Symbolic Studies." *Annual Review of Anthropology* 4: 145–161.

Turner, Victor. 1977. "Process, System, and Symbol: A New Anthropological Synthesis." *Daedalus* 106(3): 61–80.

Wacquant, Loïc. 2004. *Body and Soul: Notebooks of an Apprentice Boxer.* New York: Oxford University Press.

Walker, Margaret E. 2000. "Movement and Metaphor: Towards an Embodied Theory of Music Cognition and Hermeneutics." *Bulletin of the Council for Research in Music Education* 145: 27–42.

Walser, Robert. 1991. "The Body in Music: Epistemology and Musical Semiotics." *College Music Symposium* 31: 117–126.

Wenger, Etienne. 1998. *Communities of Practice: Learning, Meaning, and Identity.* Cambridge: Cambridge University Press.

Wetzler, Sixt. 2015. "Martial Arts Studies as Kulturwissenschaft: A Possible Theoretical Framework." *Martial Arts Studies* 1: 20–33.

Wing, R. L., trans. 1988. *The Art of Strategy: A New Translation of Sun Tzu's Classic "The Art of War."* New York: Dolphin/Doubleday.

Wong, Deborah. 2004. *Speak It Louder: Asian Americans Making Music.* New York: Routledge.

Wong, Deborah. 2008 [1997]. "Moving: From Performance to Performative Ethnography and Back Again." In *Shadows in the Field: New Perspectives for Fieldwork in Ethnomusicology*, second edition, ed. Gregory Barz and Timothy J. Cooley, 76–89. New York: Oxford University Press.

Worthing, Peter M. 2007. *A Military History of Modern China: From the Manchu Conquest to Tian'Anmen Square.* Westport, CT: Praeger.

Wrazen, Louise. 2007. "Relocating the Tatras: Place and Music in Górale Identity and Imagination." *Ethnomusicology* 51(2): 185–204.

Wrazen, Louise. 2010. "Daughters of Tradition, Mothers of Invention: Music, Teaching, and Gender in Evolving Contexts." *Yearbook for Traditional Music* 42: 41–61

Wu, Wanting. 2015. "Dancing with Lions: The Assertion and Transformation of Chinese Community and Identity in Belfast." *Queen's Political Review* 1(3): 113–121.

Yang, Fenggang, and Anning Hu. 2012. "Mapping Chinese Folk Religion in Mainland China and Taiwan." *Journal for the Scientific Study of Religion* 51(3): 505–521.

Yao, Hai-Hsing. 1990. "The Relationship Between Percussive Music and the Movements of Actors in Peking Opera." *Journal of the Society for Asian Music* 21(2): 39–70.

Yao, Haishing. 2001. "Martial-Acrobatic Arts in Peking Opera: With a Brief Analysis of Fighting Movement in a Scene from 'The Three Forked Crossroad.'" *Journal of Asian Martial Arts* 10(1): 18–35.

Yap, Joey. 2017. *The Art of Lion Dance.* Kuala Lampur, MY: Joey Yap Research Group Sdn. Bhd.

Young, Will Robin. 2006. "Southern Chinese Lion Dancing in Canada: James Lore's Martial Art Influence." *Journal of the Asian Martial Arts* 15(2): 70–79.

Yu, Henry. 2013. "Mountains of Gold: Canada, North America, and the Cantonese Pacific." In *Routledge Handbook of the Chinese Diaspora*, ed. Chee-Beng Tan, 108–121. Abingdon, UK: Routledge.

Zarrilli, Phillip. 2010. "Performing Arts." In *Martial Arts of the World: An Encyclopedia of History and Innovation*, ed. Thomas A. Green and Joseph R. Svinth, 606–608. Santa Barbara, CA: ABC-CLIO.

Zbikowski, Lawrence M. 2004. "Modelling the Groove: Conceptual Structure and Popular Music." *Journal of the Royal Musical Association* 129(2): 272–297.

Zhang, Boyu. 1997. "Mathematical Rhythmic Structure of Chinese Percussion Music: An Analytical Study of *Shifan Luogu* Collections." PhD diss., Turku University.

Zhao, Guangsheng, Chuanyin Jiang, and Yucheng Guo. 1999. "Relationship between General Physical Fitness and Special Athletic Level of Sanshou Combatants" [散手运动员一般身体素质与专项运动水平之关系]. *Journal of Shanghai Physical Education Institute* 1999(1): 67–71.

Zhou, Weiliang. 2003. *Chinese Martial Arts History* [中国武术史]. Beijing: Higher Education Press.

Index